SWEETLIGHT

THE PEYOTE BOOK
A Study of Native Medicine

Compiled and Edited by Guy Mount
THIRD EDITION

SWEETLIGHT BOOKS
Cottonwood, California

THE PEYOTE BOOK
A Study of Native Medicine

Published by SWEETIGHT BOOKS
16625 Heitman Road
Cottonwood, CA 96022

Library of Congress Cataloging-in-Publication Data

THE PEYOTE BOOK: A Study of Native Medicine
Compiled and edited by Guy Mount—Third Edition
       p.   cm.
   Bibliography: p.
   ISBN: 0-9604462-3-0   : $9.95
1. Native American Church of North America. 2. Indians of North
America—Religion and Mythology. 3. Peyote. 4. Indians of
North America—Rites and Ceremonies. I. Mount, Guy.
E98.R3P49 1993
299'.75—dc19   87-62634
                                                          CIP

**Manufactured In The United States Of America
On 50% Recycled Paper**

Dedicated to:

People Who Love The Earth

— Guy Mount

With heartfelt gratitude for the many artists, roadmen, spiritual philosophers, publishers and writers, who gave permission for their work to be included here—especially my wife and assistant editor, Jeannette—without whom, this book would not exist.

THE PEYOTE BOOK *is an ongoing, ever-growing publication. Readers are invited to submit stories, personal testimonials, research and illustrations for future editions. Please write to SWEETLIGHT BOOKS for more information.*

CONTENTS

CONTENTS

CONTENTS

Illustrations

*Contemporary Southern Plains Indian Painting: Miles Libhart, Ed. 1972
Provided by the U.S. Department of the Interior, Indian Arts and Crafts Board,
Southern Plains Indian Museum and Crafts Center: Box 749, Anadarko, OK.

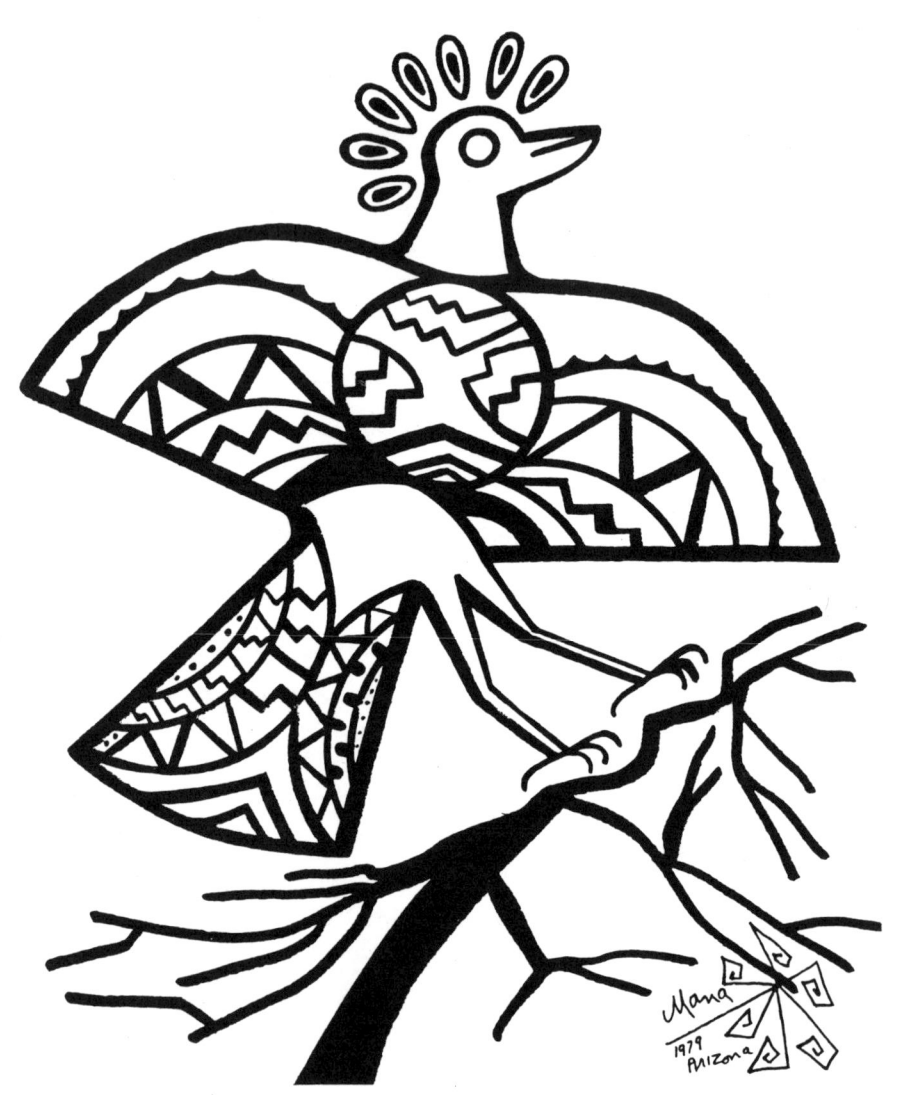

PEYOTE BIRD by Mana.
Courtesy of the Peyote Way Church of God.
Star Route 1, Box 7X: Willcox, AZ 85643

Introduction

THE PEYOTE BOOK is a collection of Native American legends, healing testimonials, spiritual and philosophical perceptions, songs, stories and artwork inspired by the "Good Medicine." These eloquent statements are found scattered throughout American Indian and Anthropological literature. It has been my pleasure to select many relevant and beautiful references to peyote and put them in one place. Scientific evaluations of peyote are also included, showing antibiotic activity more potent than penicillin, plus other medical and psychological benefits. My own studies are focused on the use of peyote in childbirth, the need for decriminalization of peyote when used as a sacrament and medicine by non-Indians, and most important—the need for ecological protection and cultivation to prevent extinction in the natural environment.

There are so many good things to say about peyote. The ancient Indian legends demonstrate the value of peyote in childbirth, and show it to be a source of physical and spiritual energy. My own four children were born at home with the help of peyote. Their mother experienced great joy, and the children were born laughing. The healing testimonials of native people suggest that the "Good Medicine" was a remedy for every illness and injury known to Indians prior to the introduction of communicable diseases by European Americans. Today peyote can help one live with incurable disorders by lifting the spirit, and it is still a powerful remedy for many serious illnesses. It is, perhaps, the most effective and sacred herbal resource on the North American continent that is available for medical self-help and spiritual enlightenment.

And yet, despite all the good things we learn about peyote, the U.S. Supreme Court has made it clear that we do not have a constitutional right to use peyote based on religious freedom. In 1990 the court decided that use of a "controlled substance" as a religious sacrament could be permitted or denied by the legislature of each state. Fortunately, the rights of Indian peyotists seem protected in most states. Furthermore, Arizona, New Mexico and New York have given all-race Churches some legal protection. I hope this book will help people in all states make educated changes in legislation, as well as their own personal lives. The laws are there to perpetuate an empire. Peyote exists to perpetuate the earth and her people.

Guy Mount,
Editor and Earthperson

Meditation

Oh great light:
come to me, come to me.
Illumine my vision
that I may see
the beauty of the world
everywhere flowing with life.
That I may hear
the sweet sound of grace,
and feel kinship with
all my relatives—
people, plants and animals,
singing together
a song of brilliant colors.

Oh Great Light:
come to me, come to me.
Let me greet you like a new plant,
all leaves open to the morning sun.

—Guy Mount

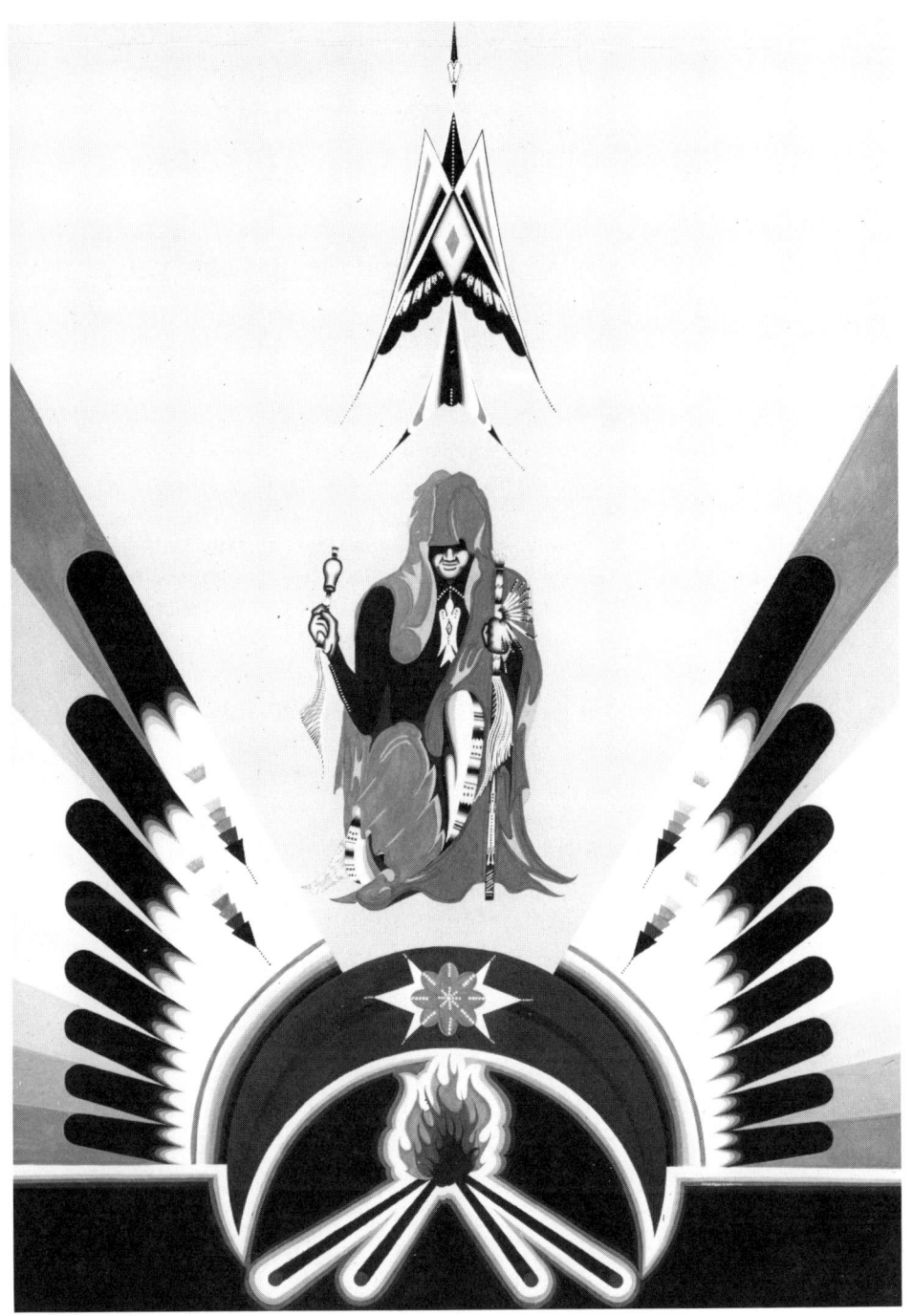

PEYOTE CHIEF (1969) By Alfred Whiteman, Cheyenne/Arapaho.
From: *Contemporary Southern Plains Indian Painting*, edited by Miles Libhart.
Courtesy: Indian Arts and Crafts Board, U.S. Dept. of Interior.

PART ONE:
Peyote Legends and Origin Stories

Many ancient legends about the origin of peyote suggest that it was discovered by women and that it is safe to use in childbirth. The Yaqui and Apache stories in Part I of this collection represent the widespread reverence and respect for the "Good Medicine", because of its compassionate benevolence toward women in distress. Several tribes in Mexico and the United States tell a story like this:

> A woman is lost in the desert. She is in labor, starving and afraid. "Something" tells her to eat peyote. Then she delivers a child easily. Her hunger is gone and her breasts are full of milk. Her strength and sense of direction return. She carries the new baby and a basket of peyote back to the people.

The special role of women and the value of peyote in childbirth is important because there is more to the "Good Medicine" than having visions. In fact, if it wasn't for the life-giving medicinal power of the plant, I doubt that peyote would have traveled from its natural location in the desert. Indian women have used peyote to relieve menstrual cramps, and the pain and suffering of childbirth, to heal vaginal cuts or infections, and to promote fertility along with the intensity of love making. Peyote can restore the vigor of elderly men and women, as well as young mothers. It is also used for divination, artistic and musical inspiration, enlightenment and spiritual encounters. Some people do have visions, but not everyone. The main characteristic of peyote is that it can heal a wide variety of disorders and promote life, as well as feed the soul.

The natural origin of peyote is in the desert along the Rio Grande in southern Texas, southward into Mexico. Ancient traders carried the "Good Medicine" to distant tribes in North and South America. The Incas used peyote to aid brain surgery, and it was a sacrament in the peaceful religions that developed in Pueblo villages along the Rio Grande.

In its natural state peyote is a small, defenseless cactus, quite abundant in places where the desert is undisturbed. It is an herb, not a drug. Drugs are manufactured by people; herbs are made by Mother Earth and Father Sun with the power of the Creator. Peyote has a mysterious connection with God, The Great Mystery, The Power of Life, or whatever you wish to call IT. This is another distinguishing characteristic of the plant: It is a healer and teacher, like Jesus, that guides our body to health and our mind to spiritual awareness. Today, the Native American Church has carried peyote to every tribe in North America. It is a major religion of Native Americans. Quite a number of non-Indians are "Friends of the Peyote Road," and would follow the Peyote Religion if it were legal in their state. We can only hope to change the heart of our people, while remaining determined to change the law.

—The Editor

A PEYOTE SONG

What if He came back,
What if He came back as a plant?
Would you let Him in,
Would you let Him into your heart?
He taught us not to fight,
He taught us to see the light,
He said that we were one
under the sun.
He sends this love to you,
He sends this love to me,
He sends this love so we
can be free.
What if He came back,
What if He came back as a plant!

—Guy Mount

How Peyote Came To People

Many years ago, my people were traveling from place to place. They went here and they went there, stopping only for a night anywhere, and going on again. They were hunting, the way...people used to. At last one woman was very tired. She was pregnant, and she lay down to rest. When she woke, her little son had been born.

The woman was frightened. The village had gone on and left her. She and her new baby were all alone in the world. She didn't know what to do. She struggled to her feet and started on in the direction she thought her people had taken.

Soon the woman grew hungry. Her child was crying for food, but until she could eat and drink herself, she could not feed the baby. She sat down beside the trail and cried with fright and desperation.

Then the woman heard a voice speak to her. "Look beside you," it said. "Pick the plant that you will find growing at your left hand. It is food and drink for all the people. Take it with you, and when you find your people give it to them. Tell them to take it with prayer, and it will heal all their ills and sorrows." The woman looked down, and there she saw a little round green cactus growing. She picked one button and scraped off the white downy fuzz that grew on it. Then she ate the cactus, and, although its taste was bitter, she felt herself growing stronger and stronger, her breasts filling with milk for the baby, and all her courage returning. When she had nursed the child, she gathered all she could carry of the green peyote cactus, and followed the trail of the village again. By nightfall, she caught up with them.

—A Yaqui Medicine Woman

AMERICAN INDIAN MYTHOLOGY: Marriot and Rachlin, 1968.
Crowell Publishers, New York.

Apache Origin Story

There is a story from long ago about the origin of peyote. It goes back to the times the Indians were fighting each other. On the other side of New Mexico a group of Indians were camped, and they were attacked by other bands. The mountains there were very high. The tribe that was attacked got scattered. There was just one woman and her boy left. They were Lipan Apaches. It was very hot and dry there. All the water had dried up. They had no food or water and there was none around them.

The woman told her boy, "I am tired and hungry and thirsty. We will rest here. Maybe I will die somewhere." It was early in the morning. The boy went out in the mountains. She told him to look around to see if he could see anyone. He walked around. Then something above spoke to him. It said, "I know you are hungry. Look down ahead of you. You will see something green. Eat it." He saw a green plant and dug it up and began to eat it. He looked around and saw many more. He ate some. Soon his hunger was gone, as if he had eaten a lot of meat. He dug some more of the plants up and took them to his mother. He told her of the voice that had spoken to him. She ate some of the plants, and felt as if she had eaten a big meal of meat. Her hunger was gone.

In the middle of the afternoon it was very hot. She said, "I do not know who gave us this. I am going to pray to him." She prayed for water and to find their people again. Later on, a cloud began to darken the sky and it thundered. Rain fell and there was water running through the mountains. They drank and rested there that night.

During the night the woman dreamed. Someone came to her and said, "Look over there and you will see a certain mountain." She looked and saw people moving along the hills. There was a creek nearby. It was east of where she and her boy were lying. In the dream she was told to go up on a high mountain in the morning and look out, and she would see her own people. She was told to take peyote to her people and a way would be made for it.

In the morning they washed and ate some peyote. She told her son of her dream. They went to the mountain and looked out, as she had been told in her dream. She saw people settling down and camping. She knew from her dream that they would be Indians. She and her boy started toward them. One man met them. He recognized them as the lost ones. They were glad to see each other. When they reached camp he told all the people about them.

The boy had the peyote with him. After they got settled the boy asked his mother to fix him a tipi, off by himself. He said he would go in that night and eat the peyote, and after that he would go into the mountains and lie down. He sat down inside the tipi and put the peyote on the ground, just as it looked when he first saw it. He prayed to the spirit that had shown him the peyote. "You have helped me. When I eat peyote tonight I want you to help me find a way for it." He had a bow and arrow, and he drummed on the bowstring with the arrow. He sang two songs. He smoked a pipe made of bone from a deer's leg. He drummed and sang all night long. Early in the morning he went to the mountains and stayed there all day and night. The following morning he came back.

He did this several times. He put up a tipi and sang and drummed all night, and then went alone to the mountains.

Soon the men began to talk among themselves. They said, "That man is doing something." One time one old man went over to the boy's tipi. He called him and asked, "Are you afraid for me to come in? I want to come in." The boy told him to enter, and the old man sat down beside him. The boy gave him the pipe and he lit it from the fire. Then the boy gave him peyote to eat.

Early in the morning they went to the mountains and returned to camp just before dark. His mother had taken the tipi down in the meantime.

After that people asked the old man what had happened.

They said they were all going into the tipi next time.

Not long afterward the boy put up the tipi again. The old man came. Another man came by and asked to enter. He was told to enter clockwise and to attend to the fire. The next morning the three of them went to the mountains and stayed until sundown. The boy's mother took the tipi down.

The next day the boy told them he was running short of peyote and would go for more. He went where it was growing and brought back more of it...As meeting after meeting took place, more men came, until the tipi was full...The others learned songs of their own, and soon everything began to fit right in the meetings. Different ones added new things...Later, Nayokogal learned of peyote and brought it to us. In time it went north into the Dakotas. To this day it is our religion. Even today different men add things to make it better. Nowadays it is held on holidays like Thanksgiving and Easter, and the feast has been added to it.

—Jim Whitewolf
Kiowa-Apache

JIM WHITEWOLF, The Life Of A Kiowa-Apache: Brant, 1969.

Good Medicine

The barefooters (Indians of Mexico) were the first to use peyote; second were the Apaches, and third the Commanches. It stayed with them a long time. Quanah Parker, chief of the Commanches, introduced it to other tribes...He went to Washington to defend the Peyote Religion. I'll say it is good medicine to use. I've been through the mill. White people usually call it mescal. Some say it is a drug; I say it ain't a drug. It is an herb. For myself I went blind. I had no hopes to see the mountains again.

So I was using this medicine. But it took a long time—I never gave up on the peyote and finally I got my sight back. I went to Oklahoma and took it with the Commanches. Some people say it makes you crazy. I know it won't. I've been taking it over thirty years and still got my head.

—Jesse Day
Wind River Shoshoni

THE SHOSHONIS: Trenholm, 1964.

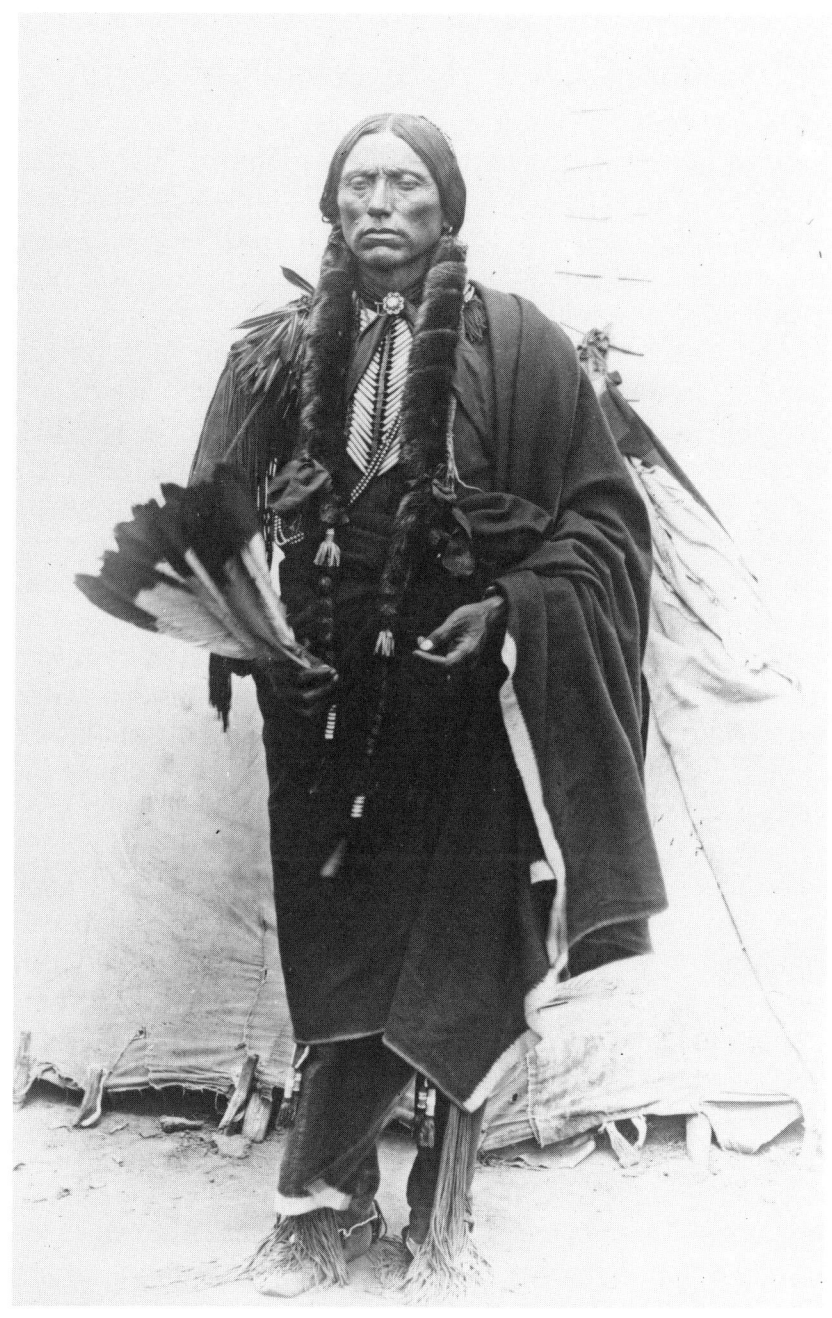

QUANAH PARKER, ca. 1891-93.
Courtesy of the Smithsonian Institution, Washington, D.C.

PART TWO:
Testimonials For Healing and Childbirth

The distinction between drugs and herbs is of great significance, because words like "drugs" and "hallucinations" to describe peyote and its effects can lead people astray. These words have negative connotations; who wants to be a "drug addict" or have "hallucinations?" That's bad and crazy. I would like to define "drugs" as man-made. Drugs are manufactured in a laboratory, or backyard still. Herbs are made by God, the Creator, Mother Earth and Father Sun. Herbs are good for people, providing they have the teachings that go with respectful use. Herbs look like plants. Drugs are found in pills, powders and bottles. Drugs can be manufactured from powerplants (like corn, barley, hops, poppies and coca), but the potent products are addicting and debilitating. The idea is to use herbs, not drugs. We are interested in having visions, not hallucinations. Peyote is such a beneficial and sacred herb that we should select words to describe it that are at least objective, if not positive. The words we use create the reality in which we live. Our self-esteem and well-being is on the line.

The biggest blessing I received from this research was to learn that peyote was valuable in childbirth. The story of "Mountain Wolf Woman" (Part 2) and the ancient legends about the good medicine persuaded me to use peyote as a birth tea for my four children. My wives insisted on it! They were listening to midwives who were experienced with herbs. Peyote has a positive reputation as a specific for childbirth among unlicensed, spiritual midwives who learned from Native American traditions. Our children were born at home, healthy and happy. Quanah smiled when I sang a birth song while the midwife snipped his cord. Ruby was born laughing. Jenny and Ben got stuck, but their mother never gave up on the medicine, and they finally came out OK.

All four births were ecstatic, more joyful for the mother than arduous. I started brewing peyote tea with the first contractions. I placed five dried buttons in a pint of water, brought them to a gentle boil, then reduced the heat to keep it brewing and hot for the mother. I gave her a sip whenever she requested. I drank some to keep my energy going. (Two buttons will give me the strength required to play a drum all night long, or paint the overhang on a house.) As the birth progressed, I gave tea, assurances and massage. We breathed together during contractions, careful to blow out all the air taken in so as not to hyperventilate. Most of the tea was gone by the time the baby came. At one point we danced around the bedroom together, joyfully laughing at "labor" during the early stage. We held hands and kissed through the greatest dilations, cried and shouted with the final pushes. Then our child was in my arms, aware and enlightened beyond me, the joyous feeling of its naked body, the glow in my heart. The eyes that looked at me and laughed, or frowned, to my birth song. Then, oh happy child squirming on its mother's stomach, lips and fingers searching to find love. Oh power of life, ever present and new! I see clearly in the birth of children that there is a power outside myself that makes everything happen. Maybe it's the spiritual material in our DNA; maybe it's God. All I know is it's bigger than me and self-evident. I call the power, "Baby Juice," because that's what this world does: it makes babies. Baby birds, baby animals, baby plants and people. Maybe even baby rocks. The power is within and behind everything. I learned that with the birth of my sweet children, and the help of peyote.

—Guy Mount, Editor

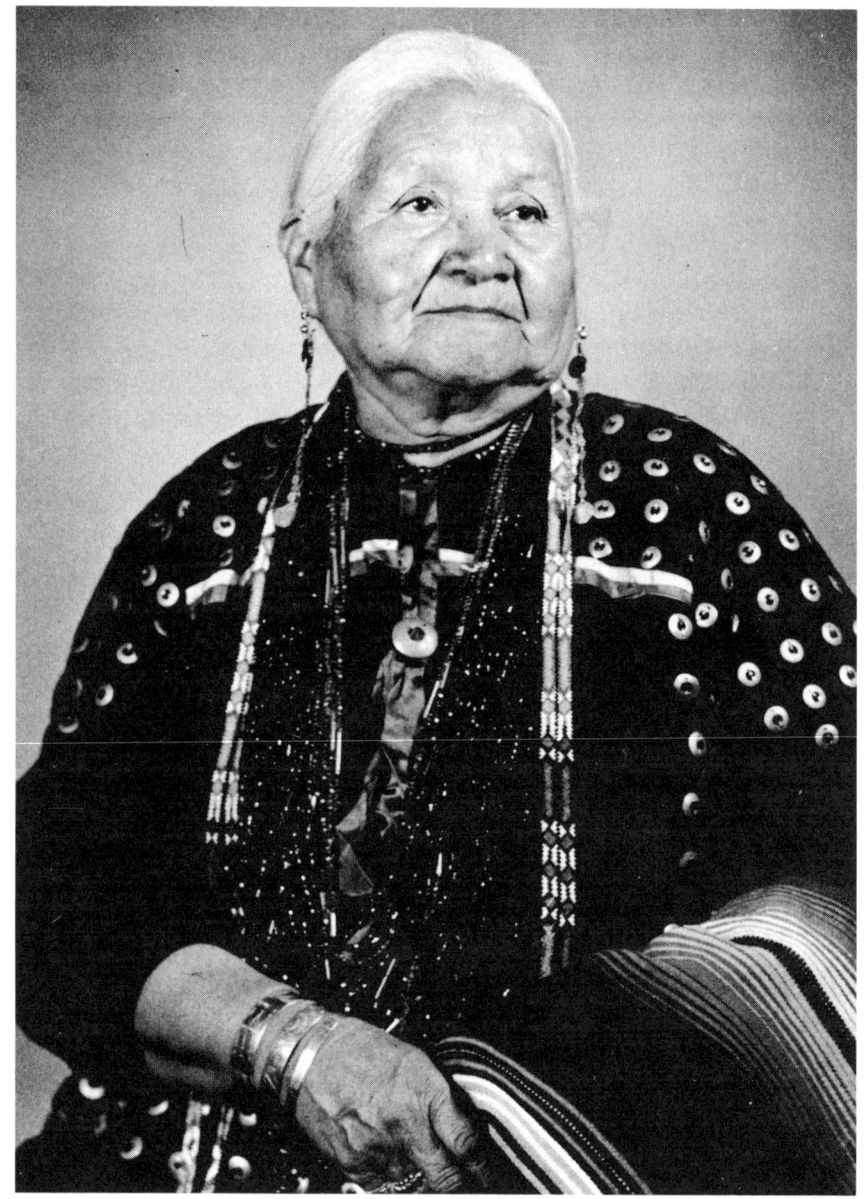

MOUNTAIN WOLF WOMAN
Courtesy the Speltz Studio: Black River Falls, Wisconsin.

I Used To Suffer

When I had children I used to suffer. I used to have a hard time and really suffered until I finally gave birth. There in Nebraska in the wintertime when we were with my sister I was about to give birth. I told her, "I think I am going to be sick." She said, "Little sister, when people are in that condtion they use peyote. They have children without much suffering. Perhaps you can do that. You always suffer so much. This way you will have it easily."

"All right, whatever you say, I will do." That was the first time I was to eat peyote. My sister did that for me. She prepared it for me and gave me some and I took it. Then I soon had the baby. I had a boy.

From that time on whenever they held peyote meetings we all attended. Mother, father, we all used to attend the peyote meetings.

—Mountain Wolf Woman

MOUNTAIN WOLF WOMAN: Lurie, 1966.

A Good Road

When I turned thirty I wanted to start a family, but was afraid of going to a hospital for such an intimate experience. In fact, I was sure that if I went to a hospital for childbirth I'd be given the wrong baby by "accident," or suffer other horrors of modern medicine. Fortunately my husband, Guy, knew a better way and we began to plan for a home birth.

On May l5, l979 at 5 p.m. my waters broke, and I knew that our baby would soon be coming. We called our midwife, Lynn, right away. While waiting for her, Guy began to fix some Good Medicine for tea. My rushes were pretty far apart at first; so I just sat around listening to music, breathing with each rush, and trying not to be afraid.

Guy said a prayer while preparing the birth tea, and now that it was ready, my turn came to say a prayer. I held the cup, and asked the medicine to help me be brave, strong and joyful. Then I sipped the tea between rushes. With each sip I felt calm and confident. As my rushes came on, stronger and closer together, I thought it was going to be too heavy to continue at home; but the "Good Medicine" saved me. I felt like I was being held in a warm, loving embrace. I knew this was right and that everything would be O.K.

Around l0 p.m. Lynn arrived. I vomited the moment she walked in the door! It was a purging. My stomach felt empty, yet full of power and strength. I continued sipping tea for 3 more hours until our daughter Ruby was born. She was shining like a light, so bright and cheerful. I was grateful that the medicine helped us have a joyful, safe birth. Ruby weighed in at 8-1/2 pounds, and she had a large head too. Lynn gave me an episiotomy, but even so she had to add five stitches due to a tear caused by the crowning of Ruby's big head. We used more peyote tea to heal the tear and prevent infection. It worked real good.

When we were pregnant the second time, a gift of Good Medicine came to us in time for the birth. My waters broke early in the morning. Guy prepared the peyote tea. We prayed together for a healthy baby. I started drinking tea with the first rushes, straightened up the house, danced around the living room, got the bed ready, played with Ruby and smooched with Guy. I "labored" fourteen hours with the birth of Jenny. The medicine helped me feel strong, happy and unafraid. I am so grateful for having found this good road for mothers and wives. It's a good road for the whole family to follow together.

—Jeannette Mount

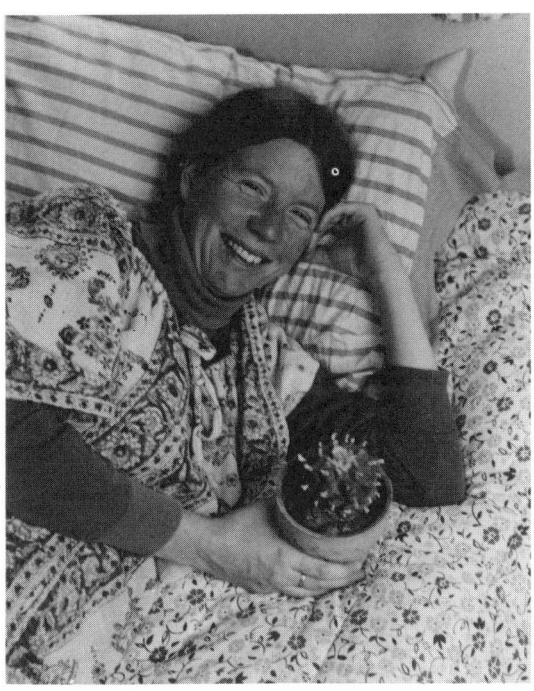

JEANNETTE MOUNT in "Labor."

Let The Medicine Do It

The doctor found something wrong with my prostate, and gave me penicillin and drugs, but I still had the same feeling. And I went to Oklahoma to see Native American Church members four years ago. There was a meeting there, with medicine, praying and singing, and boy, I felt all right again, and I brought back lots of medicine and used it at home. I would eat it and rest—up to 20, 30, 40 or 100 a day, and I seemed to be getting all right, and my bad feelings were getting out. I went back to Oklahoma again. An Oto man named Truman Dailey—we call each other brother—he wanted me to use his fireplace and way, and he gave me his ways, and I am using it that way, and I know I help lots of people. Some were sick and got helped. Some couldn't be helped. They were too far gone, and I didn't have [know] enough.

Before I couldn't work, but now I can. I worked from November until June at Piñon School. Then I had my annual leave, and I will go back Monday, and I am all right. The white doctors tried everything, at the Naval hospitals and Fort Defiance, but even though I got better for a short time, I had trouble again later on. I used the medicine every day. There is something—some part of good in this medicine...It's what you *think*. We talk to God, to our Creator, through this medicine, and in that way we get well and understand things. That's the main part...I am a Catholic myself, and I was once a helper to a Catholic priest, but through the Native American Church we don't say to *live* this way, *do* this, *know* this, we let the *medicine* do it. If we tell them that way, we might be doing it wrong ourselves, and so we don't advise people.

—A Southern Navaho Man

THE PEYOTE RELIGION AMONG THE NAVAHO: Aberle, 1966.

I Too Got Better

Seven years ago my sister's son was sick all the time. He had an earache and was having it pretty hard, and we tried Navaho ceremonies and they had no effect. My husband was worried about that and asked about the Native American Church as a possibility for the boy, and they told him how it worked, how it helped out the sick. He persuaded Mal Hancock* to run a meeting for the boy...and about midnight after the midnight water was taken out he was relieved of his pain and could hear. And in the morning it was OK. I too was sick with swellings in my joints, my arms, legs, hands, and face, and I too got better...And there was to be another meeting near Kitseely, and we took the boy with us and went to the meeting...At that meeting my swellings disappeared and I felt in better health than ever before. My husband attended a meeting at Many Farms, his third, and then a year after that they put up a meeting for him here, and we both got all right and the pains were all gone. And a couple of years later there was another meeting here. And from then on we have been doing all right.

The first time I took twenty-nine, and from then on I can't take that many. Sometimes it's hard to get, so on average, about four or five...[it gives me] a lot of pep, like when I was young. I have energy, I can move around and do anything I want to. My ailment goes away. That's the way it is.

*Pseudonym

—A Southern Navaho Woman

THE PEYOTE RELIGION AMONG THE NAVAHO: Aberle, 1966.

A Cure For Everything Bad

Many years ago I had been sick and it looked as if this illness were going to kill me. I tried all the Indian doctors and then I tried all of the white man's medicines, but they were of no avail. "I am doomed. I wonder whether I will be alive next year." Such were the thoughts that came over me. As soon as I ate the peyote, however, I got over my sickness.

Black Water-Spirit at about that time was having a hemorrhage and I wanted him to eat the peyote. "Well, I am not going to live anyhow," he said. "Well, eat this medicine soon then and you will get cured." Consumptives never were cured before this and now for the first time one was cured. Black Water-Spirit is living today and is very well.

There was a man named Walking-Priest and he was very fond of whiskey; he chewed and he smoked and he gambled. He was fond of women. He did everything that was bad. Then I gave him some of the peyote and he ate it and he gave up all the bad things he was doing. He had had a very dangerous disease and had even had murder in his heart. But today he is living a good life. That is his desire.

Whoever has any bad thoughts, if he will eat this peyote he will abandon all his bad habits. It is a cure for everything bad.

—John Rave, Winnebago

CRY OF THE THUNDERBIRD: Hamilton, 1934

Going For Peyote

About eight or nine years ago I heard of this religion around the San Juan area, and I heard so much about it, and my husband was still living, and my grand-daughter...was very sick. And a singer from around here had another patient at his home and was telling her that he had heard of this medicine in the San Juan area, and he said he was going for peyote, and so she gave him a sack of wool for the Sweetwater Trading Post. He took the wool to the store and traded it for money and went to the San Juan area. He found Ed Lyons* and bought some peyote...and I had never seen it, and two or three days later I heard there was to be a meeting at his house, and I took my granddaughter to the meeting. During that meeting I ate peyote, and they knew—those who were at the meeting— that she was sick and that she would be well, and that the best thing was to have a sing for her—Evil Way. And so they sang over her and from then on she got better. At that time on the reservation the police were looking for this peyote, and other people were scared, but I was not, because my granddaughter had gotten well on it, and so I felt it was good. And I took it ever since then. And all that time I was using it, and then my grandson became very sick, and I nursed him with this peyote, and he also got well on this medicine, and even though the police were after this medicine, so many people were getting well on it.

*Pseudonym

—A Northern Navaho Woman

THE PEYOTE RELIGION AMONG THE NAVAHO: Aberle, 1966.

This Herb

This herb here...this Peyote...this little green thing grows in the desert. There ain't no water where It grows, but It's got plenty water in It. When you eat It you ain't thirsty. It fills you up. You ain't hungry.

The whole world is in there. When I am looking at this fine little Peyote here my mind is praying. I can't think of nothing bad. All is good. It shows you everything there is to see...all the people in the world...all the different animals... all the places. It shows you all that's in the sky...everything under this earth here.

With this little Herb you can hear all the Indians in the world singing. You hear their songs and they can hear you. It makes your eyes like x-ray so you can see what's inside things. You can see inside a person and see if he is in good health or he got some sickness in there. It makes your mind like a telegram. You can send your thoughts far away to some other person and that person can send messages to you. It works like electricity. That's why when someone has this Medicine working inside them or when there's a Meeting going on somewhere people can feel It. They know it even if they is twenty miles away. They can hear the songs and feel the peoples thoughts.

The Creator put this Herb on Earth for all the people. But Indians is the only ones left know how to use it. Jesus tried to tell the white people how to use it. They forgot, I guess. They eat some kind of bread and drink wine in their church. Maybe they figured that's what He meant. But He meant this Herb...this Medicine. He was just a man like anybody, but the Creator showed Him the way...showed Him where He put Peyote on the Earth for the good of the people. That's why we got Jesus as one of the main Ones in this Indian Tipi Church. We say we have the Peyote, the Creator and Jesus. That's how we believe.

Some white people try to make laws against this Herb. They go against their own life. They don't understand It, so they don't want nobody to have It. But they can't stop It. It grows where the Creator put It. It grows in them Gardens in Texas, in Arizona and all over Mexico. There is millions of Them. Each one of Them little green Herbs is singing His own songs the Creator gave Him. Any Indian Member in good standing can hear Them all singing if he go on a run down there to get the Medicine. It is the music of the Creator put on this Earth to make the mind of humans good and clear. It is for happiness and good health.

The old Indians didn't have no books like the Bible. They didn't have no writing or no books like the white people to read and write what they believe. But Peyote is like a Bible to us here. Peyote is our Bible. When I'm with this Herb sometimes It is like a book...like turning the pages in a book. I want to know something, and I can turn to here, and here, and there. I want to know something else, so I say, "What is the meaning of that?" And then it is there...everything is in there. It is like that with the Peyote. So I think white people got one kind of book and we got another kind.

When you see this little Herb you see our Church and our Bible. If we keep on the Road It shows us we will have good life. Everything we got to depend on is right here in this Medicine the Creator give us.

—Washo Man

STRAIGHT WITH THE MEDICINE: Warren L. d'Azevedo, 1978. Heyday Books—Box 9145—Berkeley, CA 94709.

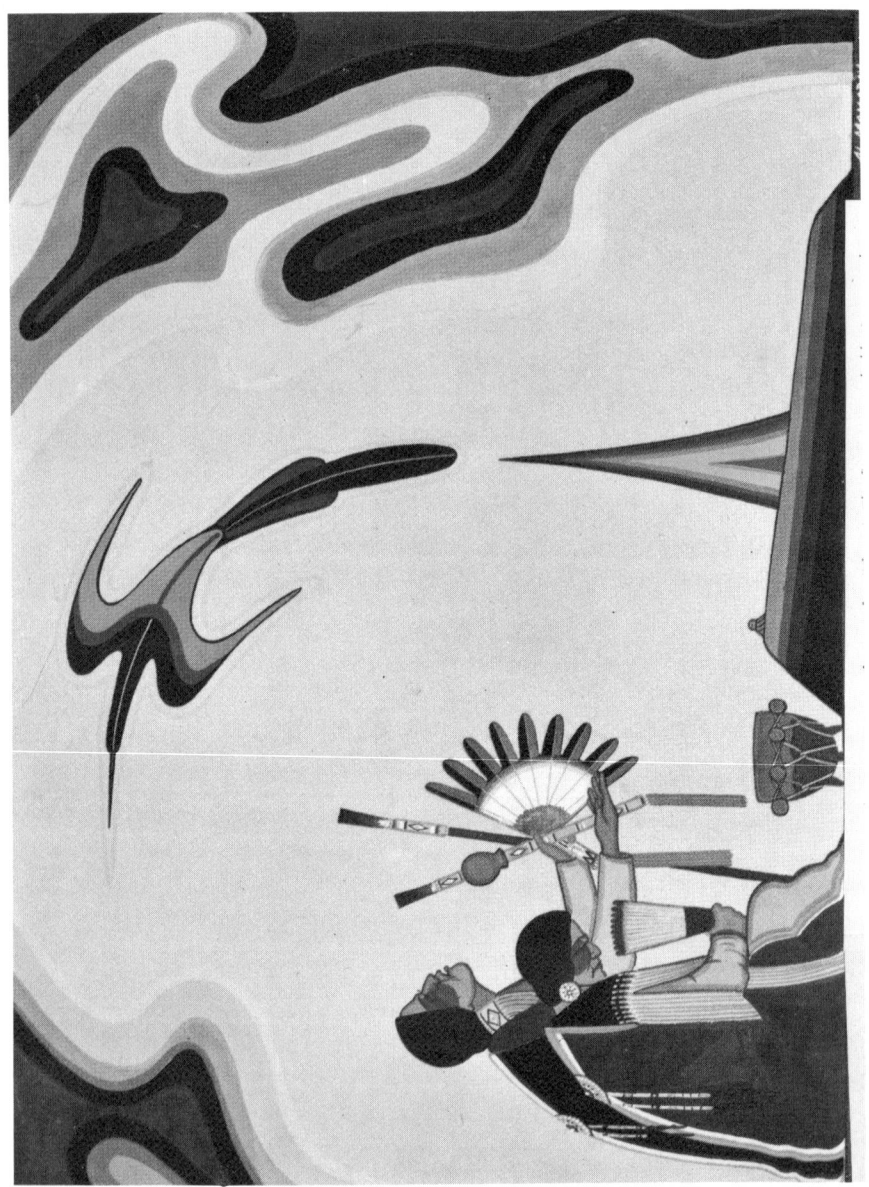

THE PEYOTE DREAMERS by Al Momaday (Kiowa).
The fire, surrounded by its curved moon of dirt symbolizes purity; the peyote bird in glorious color is the return of the spirit; the feathers symbolize the touch of the Great Mystery; the drum will beat out its signal of the concentration of the mind upon spiritual things; the peyote button (center) brings the gifts of the spirit. Courtesy Naturegraph Publishers: Happy Camp, CA 96039.

PART THREE:
The Native American Church

The Peyote Religion is a friendly road. People sit in a circle around a fire, take turns singing songs and praying, while passing around a drum, a rattle, and a basket of Good Medicine. Everyone is welcome to share their songs. The meetings can last all night, guided by an experienced Peyote Roadman. The Roadman keeps everybody on the right path. The main purposes of a meeting are to have a personal spiritual encounter, and provide a safe alternative healing center for the treatment of a wide variety of physical and psychological disorders.

Ceremonial rituals and traditions of the Native American Church will vary according to the cultural and individual influences of local chapter members. An excellent history of the Peyote Religion, showing the variety of Peyote Roads in North America, is found in the recent publication by Dr. Omer Stewart (see bibliography), and in the earlier studies by James Slotkin.

Approximately 250-300,000 North American Indians are members of the Native American Church, according to estimates by Vine Deloria and Dr. Carl Hammerschlag. There are also many non-affiliated individual followers of the peyote road, as well as established all-race religious organizations such as the Peyote Way Church of God in Arizona. I would estimate that another 250,000 non-Indians—many with mixed ancestry—would follow the peyote road if participation were legal, and access to the medicine permitted.

I believe the Peyote Road should be open to anyone who wants to follow it, regardless of race or ethnic ancestry. We are all Earthpeople, members of the same family. An Earthperson is someone who recognizes that we have a higher parentage in common—Father Sun and Mother Earth is one way to express our sense of kinship and common lineage. God and the Story of Evolution are another way of finding commonality in creation. But all these stories teach the same lesson: they reveal a kinship system that transcends cultural and biological boundaries.

Visions can transcend cultural limitations too, and the appeal of peyote to·many worshipers is that it may provide an encounter with the magical, mysterious realm that we call "spiritual" because we don't know what else to call it. If one eats enough medicine, and the situation is right—*Something Comes!* It may appear to be a person, a man or woman, perhaps it looks like an animal or bird; some people see a great light, hear music and singing, or receive other messages with personal significance. One may learn how to live a more balanced life, or how to cure a serious illness. In the Native American tradition, people are encouraged to experience the spiritual realm directly through dreams and visions. Dreams are considered the source of all wisdom.

The first time I ate peyote, I felt sick to my stomach for about an hour. Then I puked, but surprisingly it felt good to vomit—purge—what seemed to be the taste of everything bad I'd eaten in my lifetime: things like McDonalds hamburgers or Coors Beer. It seemed like bad feelings about myself and my life were vomited up too. Later on, I realized I was being shown that junk food and alcohol were making me sick, and that my life would be made healthier by giving them up.

Then I watched the fire. I felt like I'd eaten the best food in the world, better than sweet corn or steak. My stomach was full of well-being, and my heart was really happy too. I closed my eyes in contentment and was pleasantly surprised to see a light inside my own head that was even brighter and more intense than the fire. I was fascinated by the beautiful light and gave it all my attention. Then I saw faces of people coming at me out of the light. I wondered who they were and tried to recognize them, but a voice—a man's voice— told me: "Don't get attached." So I let the faces go on by.

The faces finally disappeared and were followed by images of dollar signs, green $$$ symbols, coming towards me from out of the light. I didn't feel comfortable about seeing money and tried to avoid looking at it, but once again, a voice said: "Don't get attached." So I let the money go on by until it disappeared.

Then I relaxed and concentrated on the light itself. It steadily intensified, generating a blue radiance and becoming what I now call "The Great Light." It was a living light, a loving light. It felt like the father I'd always wanted. It embraced me with warmth and good will, letting me know I was loved. Then the Light spoke to me, clearly saying: "Be cheerful and play the guitar."

I was thrilled to receive this message, because I'd been trying to learn how to play guitar for many months. When I opened my eyes and saw the fire burning and my wife sitting by my side, I felt so blessed and grateful. Then I tuned my guitar and strummed a chord. The soulful strings were a choir of enchanted voices that taught us songs and rhythms to color the night.

Since that initial experience with seven dry buttons in 1972, peyote has been my teacher, healer and benefactor. I became a real believer in 1986 when I used peyote successfully to heal the paralisis of my left arm and hand after falling from a ladder while remodeling my house. Three months after the fall, the muscles of my hand had atrophied—collapsed so badly—that I couldn't even pick up a nail or play a guitar. The doctors said there was nothing more they could do. Prescribed drugs, like Cortazone were no help. But I fianally managed to find four peyote buttons and with the help of the Light, which I could channel down my arm to the fingertips, was healed almost overnight. Thank God for peyote.

—Guy Mount, Editor

A Peyote Thought

The Peyote Man prays
to an unknown mystery
he has no name for it
                    but life.

The Peyote Man prays
to a great light
to *The Great Light*
to understand the light
                    within himself.

—Monroe Tsa Toke
Kiowa Artist

THE MAGIC WORLD, American Indian Songs & Poems:
Brandon, 1971.

Many Ways To God

The Arapahoes attribute their knowledge of the ritual to Medicine Bird (Left Hand), who, because of illness, was determined to learn about "the medicine." He is said to have gone to the Caddoes, who took him in and conducted a "healing service" in his behalf. First he was given four plants, but as the evening wore on, he continued to partake until the medicine began to fight his disease. The internal struggle caused him to weaken, but he refused to give up because he was considered one of the bravest men in the tribe. As he said of himself , "My name kept getting bigger all the time." Finally, when he had consumed a large number of plants he fell asleep and in a vision saw a special tipi with a fireplace behind which was a half-moon, which were lacking at the Caddo meeting. The entire ritual was revealed to him as he saw the way in which meetings should be conducted. The chief (as the Arapahoes call the leader of the cult) told him that he should watch carefully so that he could show it to his people. When his dream was over, he found that he had been miraculously cured of tuberculosis. After remaining among the Caddoes long enough to learn all they could tell him about peyotism, he returned to his people.

The Northern Arapahoes give William Shakespeare credit for bringing the cult to Wind River about 1895. While in school, he became seriously ill and his father sent him south in the care of White Antelope to learn about peyotism. When he arrived, he found a cult meeting in progress, but he was not permitted to enter because the tipi was already crowded. After being refused entry three times, he appeared again and was admitted. When the chief asked why he was so persistent, he explained the nature of his illness. The glands in his neck were so badly swollen that he could not turn his head.

Shakespeare was given the herbs, four at a time. As he continued to consume them and the chief prayed for him, he could feel the power of the prayers and the strength of the medicine working within him. The glands in his neck broke open and drained, and the pain and swelling subsided. After the meeting, the chief directed him to take peyote to his people and teach them how to worship. Shakespeare taught the ritual to John Goggles, who later went to Indian Territory, where he studied under Cleaver Warden, who in turn had been taught by Left Hand. Thus evolved what is known as the Arapaho Way at Wind River.

Over the years there have been various "ways," depending primarily upon the tribes and secondarily on the leaders, who have introduced their own ideas. Considering the nature of the Arapaho, it is not surprising that peyotism has had special appeal. Then, too, he is aware of the racial trend which it stresses. Peyotism through the years since its spread has served as medium of uniting tribes, at the same time generally excluding the white man, a principle to which the Northern Arapahoes are particularly receptive. Coming into prominence at a time when the precepts of the Ghost Dance had proved false, it offered consolation and an opportunity for the Indian to escape from the monotony of reservation life into an imaginary world. According to one authority on the subject, we cannot be certain that "the religion spread as a substitute for the Ghost Dance, but it is plain that it diffused rapidly around the turn of the century." He considers it in terms of accommodation.

The cult stresses a high moral code, and the priests insist that by "thinking good," one will see nothing but good, though it is not a panacea for everyone. Certain anthropologists believe that peyotism has kept down alcoholism. Unquestionably there are peyotists who drink, but probably not to the extent they would otherwise. The priests insist that if the Indian would "think right," he would not crave liquor.

Those who have unpleasant reactions or see fantastic or frightening objects during a meeting are said to have allowed their thoughts to wander. By controlling one's thinking, one finds inspiration in the quiet meditation of a meeting, where there is no dancing or hilarity of any sort. Music, a necessary part of the ritual, is subdued during the early hours, but it increases in tempo and volume after midnight, when it becomes spirited. The cult services among the Southern Arapahoes and Cheyennes became standardized through the Native American Church, with which the Northern Arapahoes are not affiliated. Each of their priests (there are about fifteen at Wind River) has his own idea of conducting the ritual, but since the Arapahoes are sticklers for form, the pattern for the Arapaho Way is more or less consistent, and it may not have changed greatly over the years.

As in the Covering the Pipe Ceremony and the Sun Dance, there must always be a vow for something of importance to the individual, to the tribe, or to the world as a whole. Vowing is a persistent pattern among the Algonquian-speaking peoples. After the vow, the Indian "puts up" the service. This suggests the pitching of a tipi, though the ceremony may be held in a house, as it is during the winter months in Wyoming. Even so, the term *tipi* is still applicable, perhaps because the cult had its origin in the south, where meetings were generally held in one the year round.

The prayer meeting, lasting from 8:00 p.m. to 8:00 a.m.., requires certain paraphernalia, namely a three-foot staff, or symbol of the authority of the chief, a ceremonial fan, a decorated gourd rattle, and a special kettledrum. Fans are symbolic of birds, messengers from Man-Above. The Northern Arapahoes favor the feathers of the eagle, prairie chicken, and the flycatcher. An impressive fan at Wind River consists of twenty-four shiny black magpie feathers, stripped halfway up the canes, which are painted white. In the center of the cluster is a Kennedy half-dollar, and added as a final touch is a scissortail feather, which, it is believed, will cause the music to resound.

The rattles are made of rounded gourds about five inches in diameter, usually with beaded handles about nine inches long. The drum, a three-legged iron kettle, is filled half full with water, into which a a dozen live coals are thrown before the well-soaked buckskin head is stretched in place. Seven lug marbles or rocks suggest the points of a star outlined on the bottom of the drum by the thong or rope which holds the head in place. Other items necessary for a meeting are a small altar cloth, a smoke stick, tobacco, corn-husk cigarette papers, a bundle of sage, and powdered cedar for incense. There is no fanfare before the meeting, no food taboo or fasting. The participants (about twenty-four in number in an ordinary meeting) assemble quietly and await instructions.* Meanwhile they talk in subdued tones, for they have come to worship, not to visit. There may be a processional, or they may merely be instructed to "go in." Within a few moments, all of the space on the perimeter of the enclosure is filled.

When the meeting opens, the chief is seated west of the altar, which has previously been arranged in the center of the circle. On his right is the drummer, and on his left is the cedarman. The sponsor, or the one who is "putting up the meeting" is on the south. On the altar there is a crescent-shaped moon with tips pointing east. A groove the full length of the top signifies the Peyote Road over which visions and thoughts pass to and from God.

The meeting opens with the cedarman offering a prayer and the chief placing "Chief Peyote" (a decorated or especially large peyote button) on the crisscrossed sprigs of sage, laid on the center of the crescent and pointing in the four directions. An impressive peyote button at Wind River is kept, when not in use, in a small, heart-shaped jewel box which has a crucifix inside the lid. Chief Peyote rests on a cushion of sweet-sage leaves. The crown of the button is painted in such a way that sun rays ("God's light") extend from the down center between

*The above discussion concerns a ceremony attended by the author at Ethere, Wyoming, on November 19, 1966. For Southern Arapaho participation in the Native American Church, see Ruth Underhill, "Peyote," International Congress of Americanists *Proceedings,* XXX (1952), 143-48. An outline of a Peyote meeting, explained by Frank Sweezy,appears in *ibid.,* 147.

pairs of tiny white tufts. On the back of the painted button is a miniature of Jesus, suggesting that peyote, like Jesus, serves as an intermediary between man and God. The Catholic influence is further noticed when some of the participants cross themselves.

A smoke establishes the mood of the meeting. A sack of tobacco is passed around and each participant "rolls his own" and takes four puffs, not for pleasure, but as part of the sacred rite. This is traditional and the only time there is a general smoke during the meeting. Sage is then passed, with each participant taking some, crushing it between his hands, and rubbing it on his body in a purification rite. After the sponsor of the meeting has explained his vow and asked that all pray for its fulfillment, he tells the chief, in detail, his need and the nature of the prayers he wishes him to offer in his behalf. Then, after the sponsor thanks all of those who have any part in the service, the chief offers a long prayer.

Cedar is put on the fire, and everyone "smokes" himself, that is, reaches out toward the fire in a symbolic gesture, then pats the smoke into his body. Next the chief starts the "peyote pan" around, and each participant helps himself to the ground substance with a spoon. The pan is followed closely by the peyote tea bucket. The participant—everyone must be one in order to attend a meeting—places the dry substance in the palm of his left hand, then in his mouth. Though the tea is as bitter and distasteful as the ground medicine, the liquid helps wash it down.

After the chief has served himself, he blows a whistle four times and a lays out the ritual items on the altar cloth. Each is smoked as it is held toward the cedar fire. Then it is raised toward heaven four times. In order, the chief, the drummer, and the cedarman hold the staff and fan in their left hand and rattle the gourd with an up-and-down motion of their right, thus setting the pattern for the participants as they sing their four songs during each of the four periods in the meeting. The drummer accompanies the chief in the first group of Opening

Songs; then the chief accompanies the drummer and cedarman as they take their turns.

The ritual items (fan, rattle, and drum) are passed clockwise, with each man present singing his allotted number of songs in turn while the man next to him accompanies him on the kettledrum. Women, if present, may hand the ritual objects from right to left, but they do not take part in the singing or oral prayers, except for the Morning Water Woman. The firechief collects the cigarette ends and piles them neatly at the points of the crescent. ("The Shoshonis have them all around," according to one Arapaho priest.)

During the singing, there is an occasional interruption by someone who wishes to offer a few words of prayer. Before praying, he smokes (four puffs) on a ceremonial cigarette. At the conclusion of his prayer, he takes four more puffs and hands the cigarette to the chief, who repeats the process, thus adding his prayers to those just offered.

Cedar is put on the coals directly east of the altar, and everyone smokes himself whenever he leaves and re-enters. Periodically through the evening, the firechief takes hot ashes to the altar as he shapes, with wood ashes, a majestic spread-eagle, with wings feather-edged with black coal dust. As one of the priests says, it is "like shaping a body," when the firechief creates his work of art with a forked stick, a brush, and his bare hands.

After the Midnight Water Songs, the firechief brings in the water and sets it before the altar. Then he smokes ceremonially, using a corn-husk cigarette, and prays. After that, he passes the smoke to the drummer, then to the cedarman, with each taking four puffs. It is then passed to the chief, who, by taking part in the smoke, adds his prayers to those offered. After smoking, the chief hands the cigarette stub to the cedarman, who places it against the crescent on the west side. The whistle is blown by the chief four times, after which the bucket is passed around and everyone drinks.

Following this, the chief goes outside and blows his whistle toward each of the four cardinal points. At the same time, four songs are being sung inside the tipi. The meeting is resumed as before with the ritual items and the peyote pan and the tea bucket making their rounds. They make four complete circuits during the course of the meeting, with each participant helping himself each time to both the ground substance and the tea. It takes a great amount of controlled thinking to overcome the nausea that results.

As the music gains tempo and the singing becomes more lively, the firechief obliterates his spread-eagle, and in its place makes a conventional ash-eagle. Better than in words, he shows the temporal nature of beauty. He collects and burns the cigarette ends which are at the tips of the crescent. Unlike the Shoshonis, who lift the smokes used by the chief over Peyote Chief and leave one leaning against the inner crescent pointing toward the chief, the Arapahoes do not go "over the top." This seems to be a fairly recent innovation, perhaps dating back to World War I.

The chief blows four loud blasts on his whistle before he sings the first of the four morning water songs. Though the words elude interpretation, the first is "like an old man talking aloud to his Creator." He is calling attention to himself. "See me—that is, take pity on me...Here she (Water Woman) comes. Pity her. Woman with water, welcome, *Ha Haa Yah.*" This is the general idea conveyed in the Water Song, which calls upon Man-Above to bless the woman and the worshipers. When Water Woman enters, she carefully places the bucket at the cross (the four directions) made between the altar and the entrance.

As the sun comes up, the second Morning Song is sung and the door is opened wide to allow the sun's rays to enter. This is told in song and alludes to the light woman has brought into the world. The other two Morning Songs are in the nature of praise and thanksgiving for the gift of water. Following the songs, the woman prays, asking God's blessing through the medium of Chief Peyote, upon the sponsor, the chief, the other leaders, the participants, and anyone else whom she wishes to include. When she has finished, the chief takes her ceremonial smoke and adds his prayer.

Breakfast, consisting of three symbolic foods—corn, meat and fruit (water is the fourth)—is passed around the circle and all partake. The first of the four Quitting Songs in the Arapaho Way suggests a group of Indians camping. They are talking in a loud voice so that all may hear. There are three other songs evoking God's mercy. As the meeting nears an end, there is a burst of music. Although the songs and prayers are nearly all in Arapaho, the spirit is unmistakable. Carl Sweezy says:

> When the service ends at sunrise, and the fast is broken
> with the water and the food that the woman (Water Woman)
> brings, those who have taken part face the day and the
> world before them with a new sense of beauty and hope and
> goodness in their hearts. Left Hand spoke the truth: There
> are many ways to God.

—Virginia C. Trenholm

THE ARAPAHOES, OUR PEOPLE: © University of Oklahoma Press: Norman, OK.

It Will Replace Christianity

The Native American Church, famed for its use of the peyote button in its sacramental worship life, has doubled its membership in the last few years. It appears to be the religion of the future among the Indian people. At first a southwestern-based religion, it has spread since the last world war into a great number of northern tribes. Eventually it will replace Christianity among the Indian people.

The largest difference I can see between Indian religion and Christian religion is in interpersonal relationships. Indian society had a religion that taught respect for all members of the society...there were no locks on doors, no orphanages, no need for oaths, and no hungry people. Indian religion taught that sharing one's goods with another human being was the highest form of behavior...

Christianity came along and tried to substitute "giving" for sharing. There was only one catch: giving meant giving to the church, not to other people.

—Vine Deloria

CUSTER DIED FOR YOUR SINS: Deloria, 1969.

It's All One

I am a road man in the Native American Church—the peyote church. I am also a *yuwipi,* a medicine man in the old Sioux tradition. I can neither read nor write. My father Henry drove off the truant officers with a shotgun. He didn't want a white school spoiling me for becoming a medicine man. When I was about thirteen years old I started out with four peyote buttons. Two years later I ate twelve buttons during a meeting. I have no book learning and don't speak good English, but I'll explain it as well as I can.

Peyote Power is the knowledge of God with peyote. God— Wakan Tanka—The Great Spirit.

We have a Bible here and the peace pipe. Some of the people coming here for this meeting are Catholics, others belong to Protestant churches, some are not even Christians and you, my friend, we haven't asked you what you believe. Because in the end, it is all the same. Jesus and Wakan Tanka are the same. God and the White Buffalo Calf Woman, yes, Christ and this stone here in my medicine bundle, the light from that kerosene lamp and the holy spirit—it's all one and the same. You get it? Eat the peyote, then you'll understand.

—Leonard Crow Dog

LAME DEER; SEEKER OF VISIONS: Lame Deer & Erdoes, 1972.AAA

A Papal Blessing

My bringing back from Rome a Papal Blessing from Pope Paul VI for the Native American Church on the Pine Ridge Reservaton, certified by a beautiful document, is also part of their history. I presented this Blessing to the members at a memorial meeting held in the fall of 1975 for one of Beatrice's sons, who had died a year before. During the midnight water call I made the following comments.

"I was in Rome as a pilgrim this summer during the Holy Year, and while there I thought of the Native American Church. And I asked the Holy Father to grant a special Papal Blessing to the Native American Church on the Pine Ridge Reservation. Pope Paul is the highest representative of Christ on earth. And he stands in a very special position between man and Almighty God. And his blessings are very powerful. They really bring down God's protecion and peace and grace when he gives a blessing. So there is a picture of Pope Paul [on the document]. And there are pictures of four churches. There are four Basilicas in Rome. Basilicas are churches that have a special position. They are considered a little more sacred than the ordinary churches. This is why they are pointed out to be Basilicas. They are churches of special grace. We know very much of St. Peter's Basilica. We all heard of that. There is also St Paul's Basilica, St. John Lateran's Basilica, and St. Mary Major's Basilica. I was able to make a pilgrimage to all four of these Basilicas and pray for the Native American Church in these special places. The thought struck me that even in Rome a person cannot get away from the four directions. One prays in the four directions even in the center of Christianity. And so the certificate says: 'Most Holy Father, Rev. Paul Steinmetz humbly begs for the Native American Church on the Pine Ridge Reservation a special Apostolic Blessing.' Then there is in Latin: 'In the year of Our Lord the Pope has granted this Apostolic Blessing in the City of Rome on June 16, 1975. That was the day the Apostolic Blessing was given.

—Paul B. Steinmetz, S.J.
A Catholic Priest

PIPE, BIBLE AND PEYOTE Among The Oglala Lakota
University of Tennessee Press, Knoxville. 1990

The Medicine Itself Will Teach Us

"...I don't believe in the idea that before a person can run a meeting, someone has to give him a fireplace. Around here, the Winnebago believe, at least I do, that the holy medicine will teach a man how to run a meeting. As you well know, in Oklahoma if a person is ever to get a fireplace, he has to spend a lot of time around a certain Roadman. Well, in my day, when I was a young man about twenty-five or so, I wanted to learn how to run a meeting. But I was very poor then, and I didn't have the money to go to Oklahoma and back here and then back there again. I couldn't afford to stay there and learn how to run a meeting.

Today in Oklahoma there are quite a few different kinds of fireplaces and different ways: the Cheyenne way, the Comanche-Kiowa way, the Commanche way, and all those others. In my day, there weren't all these different kinds of fireplaces and ways. Then, there was just the peyote way.

I don't believe that any man has to worship God in the way of another man by using his fireplace or way. Around here we believe that the herb, peyote, the medicine, will teach us how to run a meeting. Here, we just use the old simple peyote way. That's all we need. We don't need all those other different fancy fireplaces and ways with all the rules they use in your country [Oklahoma]. It's okay for Oklahoma people to have all those fancy fireplaces and different ways because they had this religion first. But up here we just need to worship God in a simple way."

—Jim Deer
Winnebago Elder

THE WAY OF A PEYOTE ROADMAN by Silvester J. Brito, 1989
Peter Lang Publishing: New York.

All My Relatives

Eleven years ago...I was very sick. And Ernie Finch* came over...Ernie boiled three peyote buttons for me, and that was the first time I saw peyote. And that day, Dan Pritchard* came and boiled nine more peyote buttons for me, and I drank that. And the medicine took effect, and I became conscious of its effects. I heard a voice saying, "This medicine is the rays of the sun and air," and under this influence I also heard that the Jewish people had written the Bible—that's how I knew about that. And I realized that there was such a thing as the Almighty. So in its teaching I found out that the medicine was used in prayer, and not often to cure, but especially for prayer, to be in communion with the Lord or Almighty.

So I figured that the purpose of the sickness was to enable me to recognize how I became sick. The teaching of the Almighty made me realize I had a father, a mother, a sister, and relatives. In the past I had not realized my position...And then I realized that my body is of earth, that I breathe through the rays of the sun and the air, and that is how I live. And I started thinking of my relatives, and I realized that the people of the world had different tongues...and names, but they are the same in having five fingers, but their skins are different. They all breathe the same air...I think a great deal of this Church.

Our bodies are of earth, and the chants are for the purpose of healing the bodies. In the Native American Church you pray for the spirit. And if a person is sick in the hospital, they give him a remedy. The remedy comes from the earth, and they apply it without speaking of God.

*Pseudonyms

—A Northern Navaho Man

THE PEYOTE RELIGION AMONG THE NAVAHO: Aberle, 1966

A Peyote Vision

In the morning at dawn
when the Water Bird fan is used
when the Water Song is sung
the priests face disappears

in its place is the Water Bird

singing

perched upon a staff
the peyote gourd beneath.

—Monroe Tsa Toke
Kiowa Artist

THE MAGIC WORLD, American Indian Songs & Poems:
Brandon, 1971.

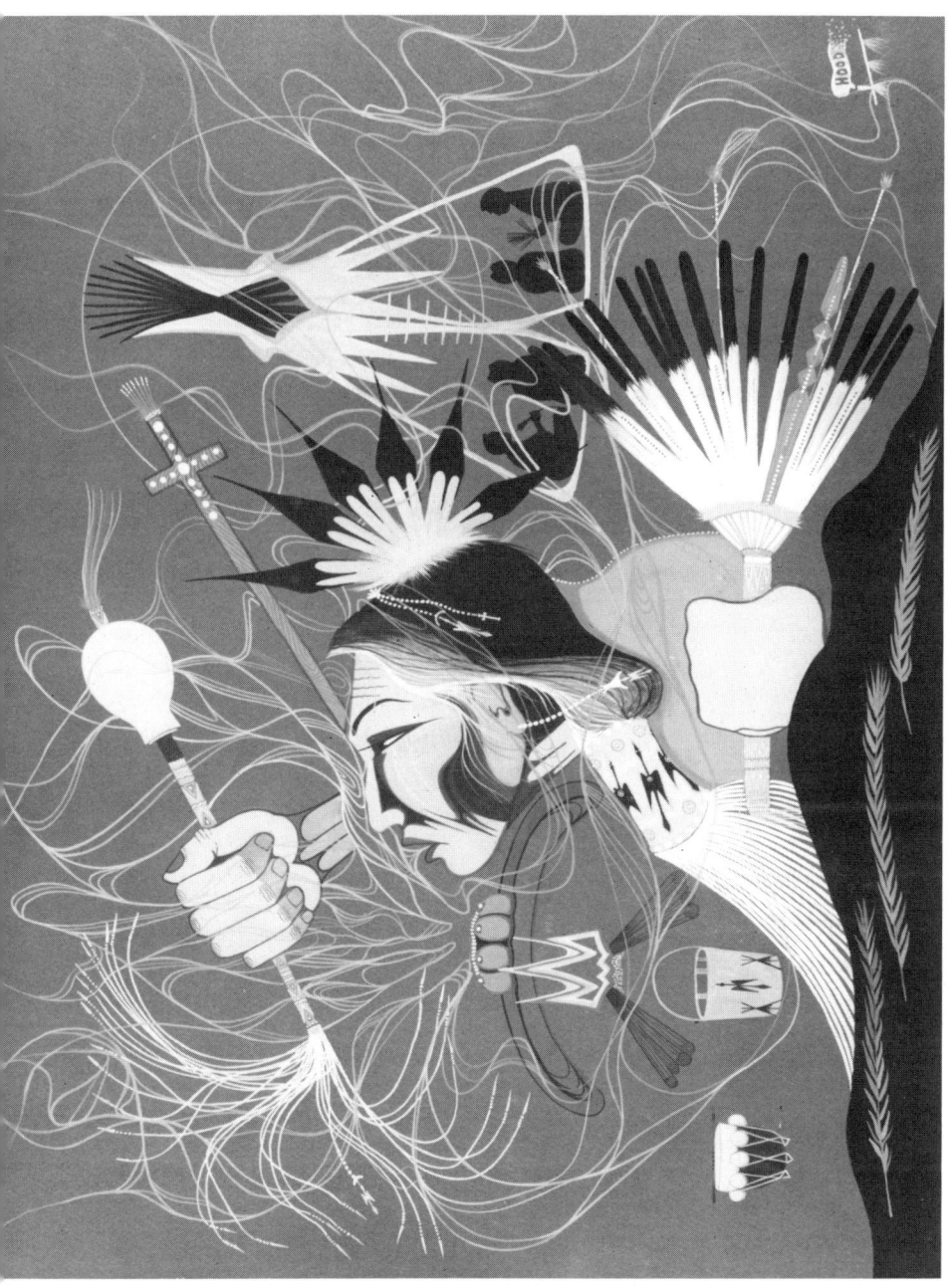

MORNING PEYOTE by Rance Hood, Comanche, 1969.
Courtesy of U.S. Department of the Interior. Indian Arts and Crafts Board,
Southern Plains Indian Museum and Crafts Center.

Four Peyote Prayers

Henry Yellowbull: "Be with us tonight. Come to us now in bright colors and sweet smoke. Help us to make our way. Give us laughter and good feelings always. Listen I want to honor you with my prayer. I want to give something, these words. Listen."

Cristobal Cruz: "Well I jes' want to say thanks to all my good frens here tonight for givin' me this here honor to be fireman an' all. This here shore is a good meetin', huh? I know we all been seein' them good visions an' all, an' ther's a whole lot of frenhood an' good will aroun' here, huh? I jes' want to pray out loud for prosper'ty an' worl' peace an' brotherly love. In jesus' name. Amen."

Napoleon Kills-in-the-Timber: "Great Spirit be with us. We gone crazy for you to be with us poor indi'ns. We been bad long time 'go, just raise it hell an' kill each others all the time. An' that's why you 'bandon us, turn your back on us. Now we pray to you for help. Help us! We been suffer like hell some time now. Long, long time 'go we throw in the towel. Gee whiz, we want to be frens with white mans. Now I talk to you, Great Spirit. Come back to us! Hear me what I'm say tonight. I am sad because we die. The ol' people they gone now...oh,oh. They tol' us to do it this way, sing an' smoke an' pray...(Here Kills-in-the-Timber began to wail, and his body quaked with weeping. No one was ashamed, and after a time he regained possession of himself and went on.) Our children are need your help pretty damn bad, Great Spirit. They don' have no respec' no more, you know? They become lazy, no-good-for-nothing drunkerts. Thank you."

Ben Benally: "Look! Look! There are blue and purple horses...a house made of dawn..."

—N. Scott Momaday

A HOUSE MADE OF DAWN: Momaday, 1966.

I Am Converted

On one occasion we were to have a meeting of men and I went...When we arrived, the one who was to lead, asked me to sit near him. There he placed me. He urged me to eat a lot of peyote, so I did. The leaders always place the regalia in front of themselves; they also had a peyote placed there. The one this leader placed in front of himself this time, was a very small one. "Why does he have a very small one there?" I thought to myself. I did not think much about it.

It was now late at night and I had eaten a lot of peyote and felt rather tired. I suffered considerably. After awhile I looked at the peyote and there stood an eagle with outspread wings. It was as beautiful a sight as one could behold. Each of the feathers seemed to have a mark. The eagle stood looking at me. I looked around in a different direction and it disappeared. Only the small peyote remained. I looked around at the other people but they all had their heads bowed and were singing. I was very much surprised...

Now since that time no matter where I am I always think of this religion. I still remember it and I think I will remember it as long as I live. It is the only holy thing that I have been aware of in all my life.

—A Winnebago Man

THE AUTOBIOGRAPHY OF A WINNEBAGO INDIAN:
Radin, 1920.

Using Peyote Right

Rolling Thunder had told us at Council Grove that he was a member of the peyote religion, and since then I had learned from him some appreciation of the rituals. He considered these affairs "serious business." "It's a purification ceremony," he had said, "like most of our ceremonies. It's not used to get high or for foolishness. It's used in a way that we want to cleanse our systems, and our minds, so we can put ourselves on a higher plane of life." Rolling Thunder said he knew that there were a couple of groups of white people now who are using it right, "but the great majority of them aren't using it right at all, and they might be punished for it. I've seen some of the results of punishment...It's terrible when it kicks back on you. But peyote is good. I've seen it used for many good purposes when it is used right."

—Rolling Thunder

ROLLING THUNDER: Boyd, 1974.

A White Peyote Church

The peyote Indians are nonviolent people. In fact one of the famous peyote chiefs was called Quanah Parker—the town of Quanah, Texas, is named after him. Quanah Parker was a famous war chief at first, and he was dedicated to the principle that the only good white man was a dead one. He had more scalps, personally, than all the rest of the war chiefs of that tribe put together, and he renounced violence after his first peyote trip. The peyote Indians are nonviolent. He became one of the most famous peyote road chiefs after that; after having been a war chief he became a road chief. Another nice thing about peyote, by the way, that's interesting, is that as well as the American Indian peyote churches there are black peyote churches, because there used to be tribes of runaway slaves. Enough of them would run away till there would be enough of them together to be a tribe, and some of them got to be peyote Indians. They became like black Indians. And there were and are peyote road chiefs, black ones, Indian ones, and a white one too, that I know about—this one.

—Stephen Gaskin

THE CARAVAN: Gaskin, n.d.
Courtesy of The Book Publishing Company
C/O The Farm—Box 180—Summertown, TN.

The Church Of Father Peyote

The first time I attended the church of Father Peyote, I got quite sick—and I was only sitting outside listening to the music. They passed some tea around. I tried it and became violently ill.

I thought that was the end of my relationship with Father Peyote. There was no way that I would sit up all night just to get sick. On that first visit to a Native America Church meeting in 1965, I did not realize that the process it offered was not to be taken lightly. It took me ten years to make a return visit, but now the church has become a place of healing and enlightenment for me.

To the believer, peyote constitutes a sacrament, not a drug. Peyote has absolutely no recreational aspects for the church participants. You must come to peyote as to truth, in an attitude of worship.

Let me explain at the outset that in matters of the Peyote Church, I am a guest who has come to dinner; that does not make me an expert on the entire family. I know what I have seen, and there is much I don't know. I go as a fellow traveler. I don't bring friends to observe the colorful ritual. This is a sacred time to me and to every other participant in the service.

The most spiritual place I know is the tipi of the Peyote Church. I used to go to synagogue on the high Jewish holidays, but I can no longer feel the presence of the spirit in a group larger than forty.

Indians have a very different concept of where you worship. The whole Earth is the temple. Any place you stand is a church. The tipi is a nestling enclosure on the Earth Mother's breast, a place of sharing among a small group. Here each can worship at his or her own time, as the heart directs, in his or her own language.

I sing my Jewish songs in the tipi, and I wear my father's prayer shawl, the one he wore at his bar mitzvah in Germany.

My Indian friends say that it does not matter in what language you sing; there are always at least two people who understand— you and the Creator.

The first time I sat before the coals in the tipi, I saw crematorium ashes. I do not see them as such anymore. I have allowed myself to become liberated. I understand that I am flawed and imperfect, so it's okay to feel small and weak. I am freer of the domination of those fears.

The more you work with the mind, the more you realize you can't know it. The more you seek to touch your spirit, the more you realize that you must enter some altered state of consciousness to burst free of the conventional limitations of flesh and rationality. This is what the Peyote Church is about.

—Carl A. Hamamerschlag, M.D.
Psychiatrist and Teacher
Phoenix, Arizona

THE DANCING HEALERS: Hammerschlag, 1988.
Harper & Row, San Francisco

The Peyote Road

The Peyotist ethical code constitutes a way of life called the "Peyote Road," and conforming to the ethic is called "following the Peyote Road." This ethic has four main parts:

a. Brotherly love. Members should be honest, truthful, friendly and helpful to one another. This is conceived as a spelling out of the Golden Rule.
b. Care of family. Married people should not engage in extra-marital affairs, and should cherish and care for one another, and their children. Money should be spent on the family as a whole, rather than selfishly.
c. Self-reliance. Members should work steadily and reliably at their jobs, and earn their own living.
d. Avoidance of alcohol. There is a maxim, "peyote and alcohol don't mix."

The Peyote Road is learned in various ways. The beginner learns about the code informally from older members. Some tribes include within the rite the formal preaching of ethical doctrine. But most important of all, after one eats Peyote the Peyote itself teaches him what should or should not be done, either by ethical revelation in a vision, or by sensitizing his conscience. This is summed up in the maxim, "Peyote enlightens your heart and mind."

—James Slotkin

THE PEYOTE RELIGION: Slotkin, 1956.

Medicine People

My experience with the army forced me to figure out who I was. In that way it was good medicine.

Moving down the road, I decided it was time to learn more about my people, so the early 1950's became a time of learning, expanding, and studying the medicine of many Native American brothers and sisters.

I traveled through North Dakota, earning enough money to buy a car, then left for Omaha, Nebraska. When I arrived there, I was broke, and ended up on skid row (16th Street), where a lot of other Indian people were staying. Finally, I landed a job with a Hinky Dinky wholesale market, and there I met some Winnebago brothers. After a few days they invited me to come to a peyote ceremony. I'd heard much about the Native American church, the peyote religion, but had never experienced it firsthand.

The first night that I was supposed to go, I couldn't make it. They set up a spot on the floor for me anyway, and drummed all night to the empty seat. The following week I was again invited to go and that time I went.

Meetings were held in the house of Ballantine Parker, an Omaha Indian who was the local leader of the Peyote church. I brought him a wallet as a gift.

Both Winnebago and Omaha Indians were there. The ceremony began at about nine in the evening, and lasted until dawn.

The room was bare; the furnishings had been taken outside. We all sat down on the floor. There was a woman in the room, and Ballantine Parker introduced her.

"This sister is very sick," he told us, "and she's asked us to pray for her."

A young man, called the "servant of the peyote," brought in a pan of hot coals and placed them in front of Ballantine who took cedar and tobacco, and offered it on the coals, making prayers.

I could feel the power rush into the room.

Now the servant came into the room with a cloth bag; it was filled with dried green peyote buttons, the sacrament of the peyote religion. The buttons were passed to everyone, in a sunwise manner. I took two, broke them open. Inside, there was a cottony substance which had to be removed.

We began to chew the peyote buttons; they tasted like bitter chocolate, only stronger. After we'd finished eating them, the servant brought us peyote tea.

A friend of mine, Hawk John, began to sway and chant; a man beside him beat a drum while Hawk John sang four chants. He held a rattle and a beaded staff in his hands which the people call the staff of life.

Others began to sing. Some chanted; some just prayed, and the peyote sent us on a journey. It was a feeling of great expansion, a buzzing, a beating inside the center of the forehead.

When Hawk John finished his four chants, he passed the staff of life to the next man, sunwise. This was the way of the ceremony; each man would take the rattle and staff, and chant or pray. The man beside him would beat the drum in accompaniment.

The peyote filled me, gave me a sense of depth and dimension, a sense of opening, of oneness with the universe. Everything, the beadwork, the room itself, the faces of the others, grew visually intense; every detail came into focus. I became an eagle, soaring with the chant, over a lake of clear blue water. My veins filled with love, and the drumbeats entered, became one with my pulse.

The Great Spirit was everywhere. Time had stopped and we were ancient beings, without need of language.

After awhile, Ballantine Parker spoke.

"Me and my wife," he said, "are happy to share this meeting with our Winnebago brothers. We use tobacco and cedar here tonight, to honor both ways. And we welcome our Chippewa brother." He nodded at me.

The staff passed around the circle three times that night. It must go completely around, no matter how late it gets.

Some brothers prayed for loved ones in prison or hooked on alcohol; some praised the peyote for its healing power, for its vision.

The woman who had come to be healed seemed to be much better.

In the morning, we shared a ceremonial breakfast...first came a bowl of water, again passed sunwise. Each person took a drink, and thanked the Great Spirit for the water's gift of life. Next, corn was passed and we all ate from a common bowl, again thanking the Creator. The corn was symbolic of all grains on Mother Earth. Next, peaches were passed around, representing all the fruits and berries, and finally we ate from a bowl of meat. Each dish, again, represented a separate kingdom of foods, which the Great Spirit had provided on the Earth Mother for us.

After this breakfast, we visited for several hours and then, at noon, we had a peyote feast. This meal signified the ending of the ceremony.

The peyote meeting was a meeting of hearts; all things had been done with love and humility. At other peyote meetings, which I've attended in California, the brothers would light a cornhusk cigarette filled with tobacco, to make a prayer. They would pass it around, each praying first in English, then in their Native language.

The first meeting, with Ballantine Parker, was a very powerful experience. Nobody celebrates peyote just to get high, or go tripping; the peyote brings power and energy into you. And what really brings power to that medicine is the all-night beating of the drum; you can hear it in your head, feel it pounding in your chest, for three weeks afterward.

The drum in a peyote meeting is a special kind; it's a small kettle drum that you can pick up and hold. Around the sides of the kettle there are seven small stones, and around each of the stones, the buckskin top is wrapped. The stones are wrapped with thong to stretch the hide tight, first, in a circular line, then up and down across the bottom of the kettle. When wrapped right, the thong forms a seven pointed star across the bottom of the drum.

The Kettle is filled with water and when the drum has been beaten for about an hour, the hide "opens up"; that means its resonance improves. There is the beating sound then, like a heartbeat, and the whirring, reverberating sound as vibrations travel through the water. Sometimes, when the ceremony has been underway for a long time, the water in the kettle evaporates. When it does, you suck hard against the buckskin, thus creating a vacuum in the kettle; then you pour more water onto the hide. It goes right through, refilling the kettle.

Like your heartbeat, the drum becomes a part of you; it carries you, over and over. And people do change into animals sometimes, like I did, into an eagle. Castaneda's pretty accurate, in the Don Juan books; you can change into a crow, or a coyote, with peyote or other herbs, or without them.

The peyote is a healer both spiritually and physically; it has a quinine effect. I've made peyote tea for some of my people when they're feeling sick, and it always helps them. It's good medicine, but it is a sacrament and, I feel, should only be used ceremonially under the direction of people who have been properly trained in its use. Otherwise you don't get the full power of it. Taking it by yourself isn't the same, and I don't recommend it as a thing to play around with.

—Sun Bear

THE PATH OF POWER: Sun Bear, Wabun & Barry Weinstock, 1987. Available from: Bear Tribe Publishing-Box 9167-Spokane,WA 99209.

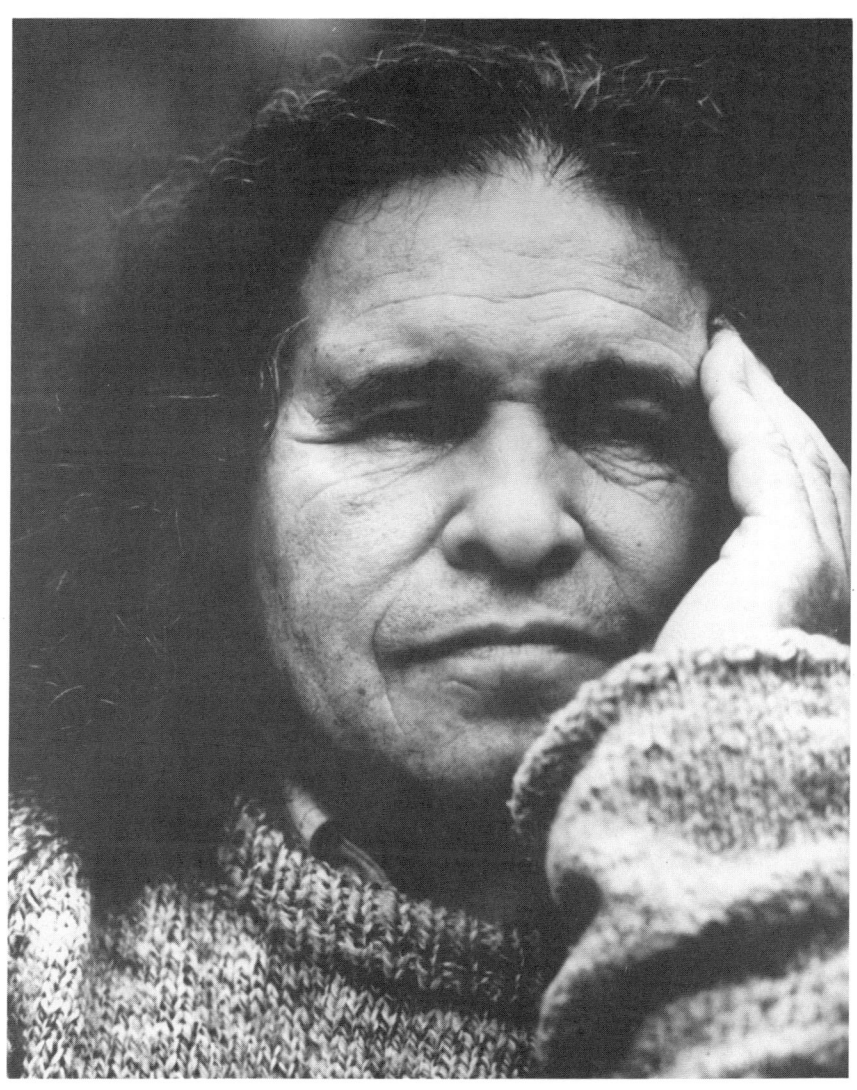

SUN BEAR
Courtesy of The Bear Tribe, East Coast Office.
Box 199: Devon, PA 19333

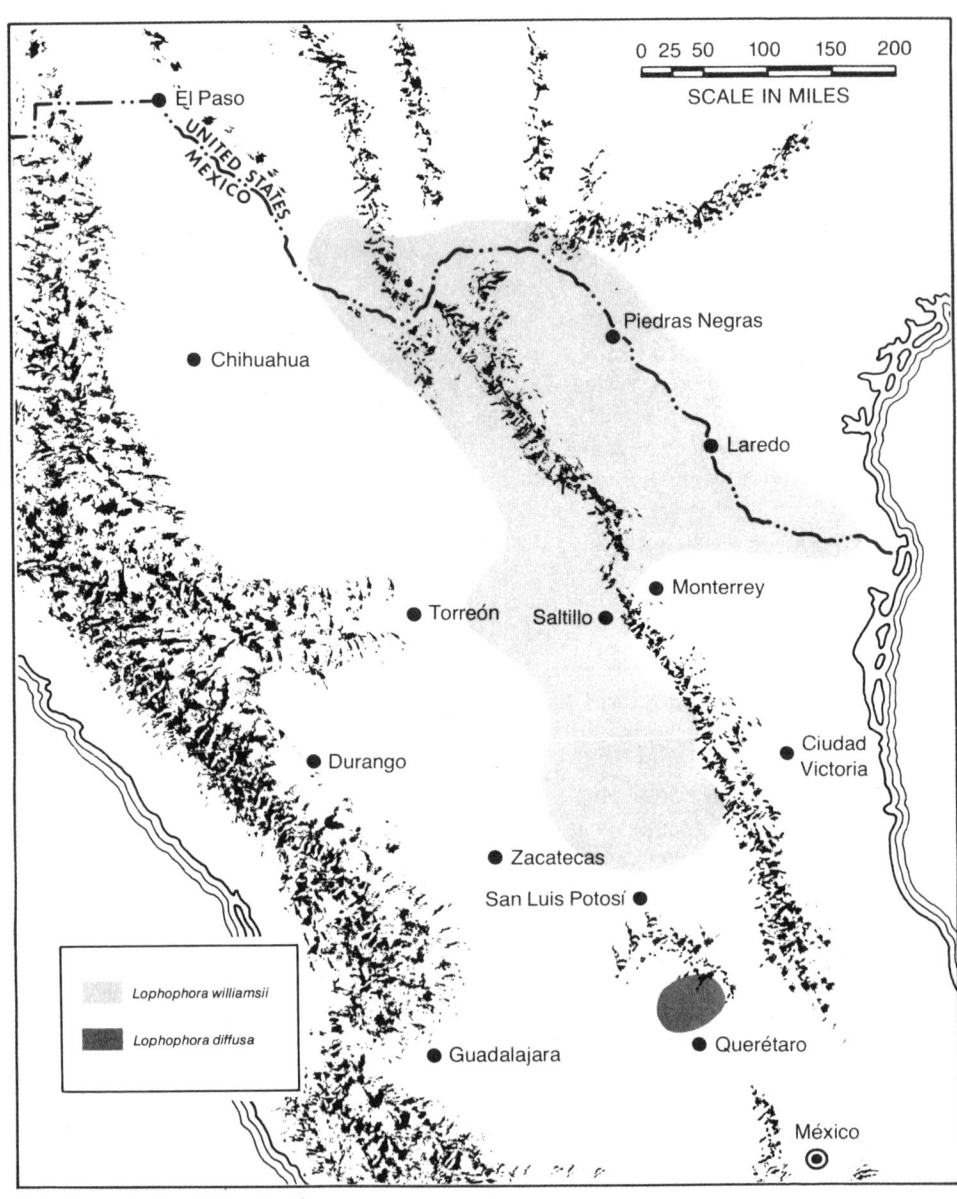

Natural distribution of the two species of peyote, *Lophophora williamsii* and *L. diffusa,* by E.F. Anderson, 1980.

PEYOTE, THE DIVINE CACTUS: University of Arizona Press, Tucson, AZ.

PART FOUR:
Gathering Peyote

People have been gathering peyote in the desert for thousands of years. It was quite abundant in southern Texas until the desert was spoiled by modern dry-land cattle ranching techniques and the development of oil wells. Today land along the Rio Grande is being turned over by disc-plows 20 feet wide pulled by giant Caterpillar Tractors. The plows dig to a depth of two feet and bury all the bushes, cactus, turtles and other things that made a living desert. The ranchers plant buffalo grass and create a vast pasture, level and even, like a cemetery lawn. Peyote is disappearing at the rate of 20 acres an hour where these plowing machines operate. The development of oil wells with gravel roads and storage facilities account for additional habitat degradation and loss of medicine. In fact, much of the land in Starr County, Texas (where peyote used to grow as thick as daisies in a pasture field) is now controlled by Oil Companies. Therefore it is important that we harvest peyote even more carefully and reverently. It may soon be gone forever in the United States unless steps are taken to establish a peyote nature preserve, and decriminalize commercial cultivation. (It was legal to cultivate and sell peyote through the mail until 1972 when President Nixon started a "War on drugs." Federal agents were sent to confiscate plants from green houses along the Rio Grande.)

When gathered properly, peyote roots will generate new crowns the following season. The plant should be cut off above ground level, not dug up. The open wound should be sprinkled with sulfur powder or charcoal dust to prevent infection. The rootstock will continue growing and produce new buttons for other pilgrims.

They say it is "good luck" to take the family along when searching for peyote. That's how I found it, or rather it found me. My son, Quanah, was five at the time. Ruby was still nursing, so she stayed with Jeannette near our car which was parked off the road in Starr County, Texas. Quanah and I walked away from the car, following a cattle trail through the mesquite and prickly pear. Quanah was barefoot, running here and there. Suddenly he ran down a side trail and disappeared! I trailed behind, shouting his name and telling him to "stop." But he kept going, and I had to crawl under a thornbush, annoyed because I thought my son was distracting me from the serious pursuit of peyote.

I was carrying Quanah's tennis shoes, so the first thing I looked at when I found him in a little clearing on the other side of the thornbush was his feet. I wanted to be sure he hadn't picked up a cactus spine, but his feet were safe enough; he was standing on a clump of peyote! I was still on my hands and knees, close to the earth, and could see peyotes growing under all the bushes and outgrowths of larger cacti. I started giving thanks and singing a medicine song.

"Look, Dad!" Quanah said. "A Turtle."

Indeed, a desert tortoise was buried in the sandy soil and pebbles up to his rear end. We could see his tail and hind legs. The turtle was busy eating the succulent roots of a peyote plant. I suppose that was the major source of food and water for miles around. The turtle was obviously content, and I imagine very wise. It had been on this earth longer than me, and showing by its own existence the merits of the medicine.

—Guy Mount, Editor

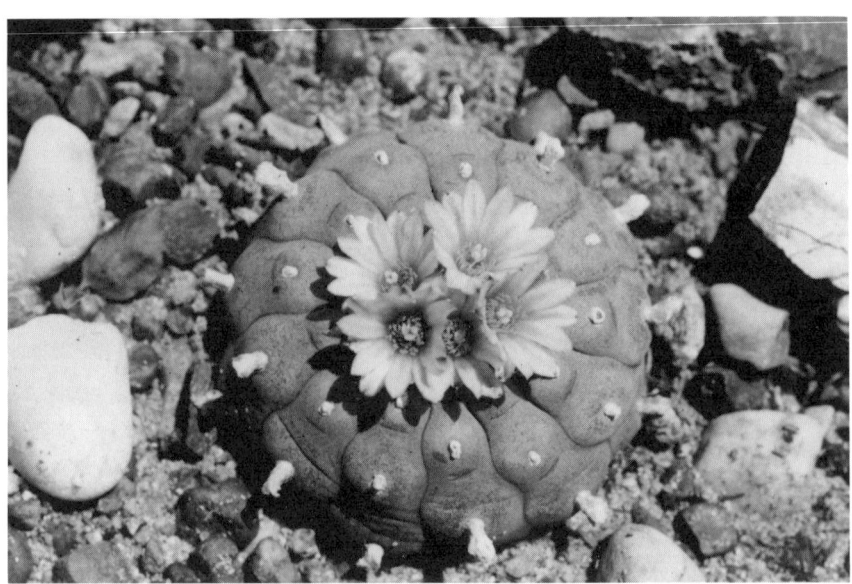

PEYOTE IN BLOOM, courtesy of Larry Noggle.

A Big Blessing

It was summer...Not the best time to gather peyote, but the only time we had. My husband had his vacation then, and the kids were out of school.

We took my brother and both sisters, and the children's adopted grandfather, and the children, of course. That made a carful! When we got down below Fort Stockton, Texas, we found a clear place with a little spring, and got out and made camp for the night. There were a lot of bushes with lavender flowers hanging from them in bunches, but we'd never seen those flowers so we didn't pay much attention to them. We just camped near the spring and cooked and ate our supper, and went to sleep.

In the morning, when we had all washed ourselves, grandfather took out his old stone pipe and filled it. Then he blew smoke to the four corners, and down to our Grandmother the earth, and up to the Above One in the sky. He prayed strong. He prayed real good. And he went on and on, praying and praying, and nobody wanted to say anything, but we were all getting pretty hungry.

My daughter was about seven then, and she just plain gave out, the way kids do. Finally she stretched out on the ground, and sort of dozed off under one of the big lavender bushes.

Then Grandpa stopped praying, and all at once I heard Jeanne say, "Mama what's this thing?" She was pointing to a little low green plant, close to the ground, right by her hand. "Why, I'm sitting on some," she said, and jumped up, and there they were! Peyotes all over the place, like you never saw them grow. Grandpa said it was a big blessing, that a little girl had found them.

—A Sac and Fox Woman

PEYOTE: Marriott and Rachlin, 1971.

The Gathering Of Peyote

When a man goes out to gather peyote, he stops before taking any and prays. Then sometimes he sings peyote songs right in the middle of the field. Among the Indians, when they pray at this time they first take out a cigarette and pray with the smoke...When the peyotes are growing, there will be a big one with several little ones around. They cut off the tops without bothering the roots. The plants are not dug up...

Peyote is pretty hard to find when you are looking for it. A person who has been there picking it before finds it easily, but a person who has not used it does not recognize it though he is in the middle of a whole clump of peyote. Once he sees one, another appears and so on till they all come out just like stars.

If you are having a hard time finding them, you do this. When you find just one by itself you eat it. When it takes effect, when you get a little dizzy, you will hear a noise like the wind from a certain direction. Go over there. You will find many of them. From the place where the noise is coming you will get many peyote plants.

—An Apache Man

AMERICAN ANTHROPOLOGIST: "The Use of Peyote by the Carrizo and Lipan Apache Tribes," Vol. 40:271:Opler.

A Peyote Gathering Song

What pretty hills, what pretty hills,
So very green where we are.
Now I don't even feel,
Now I don't even feel,
Now I don't even feel like going to my rancho.
For there at my rancho it is so ugly,
So terribly ugly there at my rancho,
And here in (Peyote Country) so green, so green.
And eating in comfort as one likes,
Amid the flowers, so pretty.

Nothing but flowers here,
Pretty flowers, with brilliant colors,
So pretty, so pretty.
And eating one's fill of everything,
Everyone so full here, so full with food.
The hills very pretty for walking,
For shouting and laughing,
So comfortable, as one desires,
And being together with all one's companions,
Do not weep, brothers, do not weep.
For we came to enjoy it,
We came on this trek,
To find our life.

For we are all,
We are all,
We are all the children of,
We are all the sons of,
A brilliantly colored flower,
A flaming flower.
And there is no one,
There is no one,
Who regrets what we are.

—Huichol Song

FLESH OF THE GODS: To Find Our Life, Peyote Among The Huichol Indians of Mexico. Furst, 1972.

Chew It Well

When every one of the companions had chewed a piece of the first sacrificial peyote, Ramon took out his fiddle and one of the others a quitar (both homemade), and the veterans stood aside in a group to sing and dance...In the meantime, another gourd had been filled with peyote cut into small pieces, and the initiates were not allowed to rise until they had emptied it. As the bowl was handed around, the others, led by Ramon, exhorted them over and over to "chew well, companion, chew well, for that is how you will see your life." Lupe then took a sizable whole plant, sliced off the bottom, lifted her long magnificently embroidered skirt, (like Ramon's clothes, it had been specially make for this journey) and rubbed the moist end of the cactus on her legs, especially on the numerous small scratches and cuts inflicted by spines and thorns during the trek through the desert. The others followed her example. Lupe explained that peyote not only discourages hunger and thirst and restores One's spirit but heals wounds and prevents infection.

—Huichol Pilgrims

FLESH OF THE GODS: To Find Our Life, Peyote Among The Huichol Indians of Mexico. Furst, 1972.

Peyote Dancing

The Tarahumara Peyote dance may be held at any time during the year for health, tribal prosperity, or for simple worship. It is sometimes incorporated into other established festivals. The principal part of the ceremony consists of dances and prayers followed by a day of feasting. It is held in a cleared area, neatly swept. Oak and pine logs are dragged in for a fire and oriented in an east-west direction. The Tarahumara name for the dance means "moving about the fire," and except for Peyote itself, the fire is the most important element.

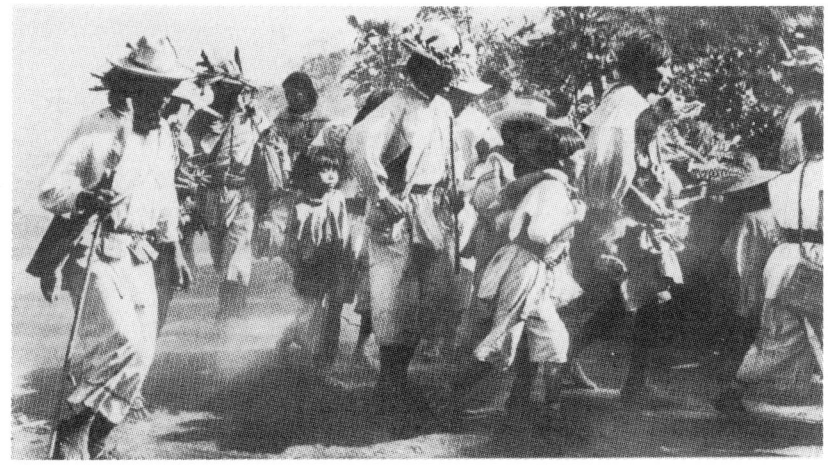

HUICHOL DANCERS: Courtesy of Richard E. Schultes.

The leader has several women assistants who prepare the Hikuri plants for use, grinding the fresh cacti on a metate, being careful not to lose one drop of the resulting liquid. An assistant catches all liquid in a gourd, even the water used to wash the metate. The leader sits west of the fire, and a cross may be erected opposite him. In front of the leader, a small hole is dug into which he may spit. A Peyote may be set before him on its side or inserted into a root-shaped hole bored in the ground. He inverts half a gourd over the Peyote, turning it to scratch a circle in the earth around the cactus. Removing the gourd temporarily, he draws a cross in the dust to represent the world, thereupon replacing the gourd. This apparatus serves as a resonator for the rasping stick; Peyote is set under the resonator, since it enjoys the sound.

Incense from burning copal is then offered to the cross. After facing east, kneeling, and crossing themselves, the leader's assistants are given deer-hoof rattles or bells to shake during the dance.

The ground-up Peyote is kept in a pot or crock near the cross and is served in a gourd by an assistant; he makes three rounds of the fire if carrying the gourd to the leader, one if carrying it to an ordinary participant. All the songs praise Peyote for its protection of the tribe and for its "beautiful intoxication."

As with the Huichol, healing ceremonies are often carried out. The Tarahumara leader cures at daybreak. He first terminates dancing by giving three raps. He rises, accompanied by a young assistant, and circling he patio, he touches every forehead with water. He touches the patient thrice, and placing his stick to the patient's head, he rasps three times. The dust produced by the rasping, even though infinitesimal, is a powerful health and life-giver and is saved for medicinal use.

The final ritual sends Peyote home. The leader reaches toward the rising sun and rasps thrice. "In the early morning, Hikuli had come from San Ignacio and from Satapolio riding on beautiful green doves, to feast with the Tarahumara at the end of the dance when the people sacrifice food and eat and drink. Having bestowed his blessings, Hikuli forms himself into a ball and flies to his shelter at the time."

—Richard E. Schultes

PLANTS OF THE GODS: Schultes and Hofmann,1979.

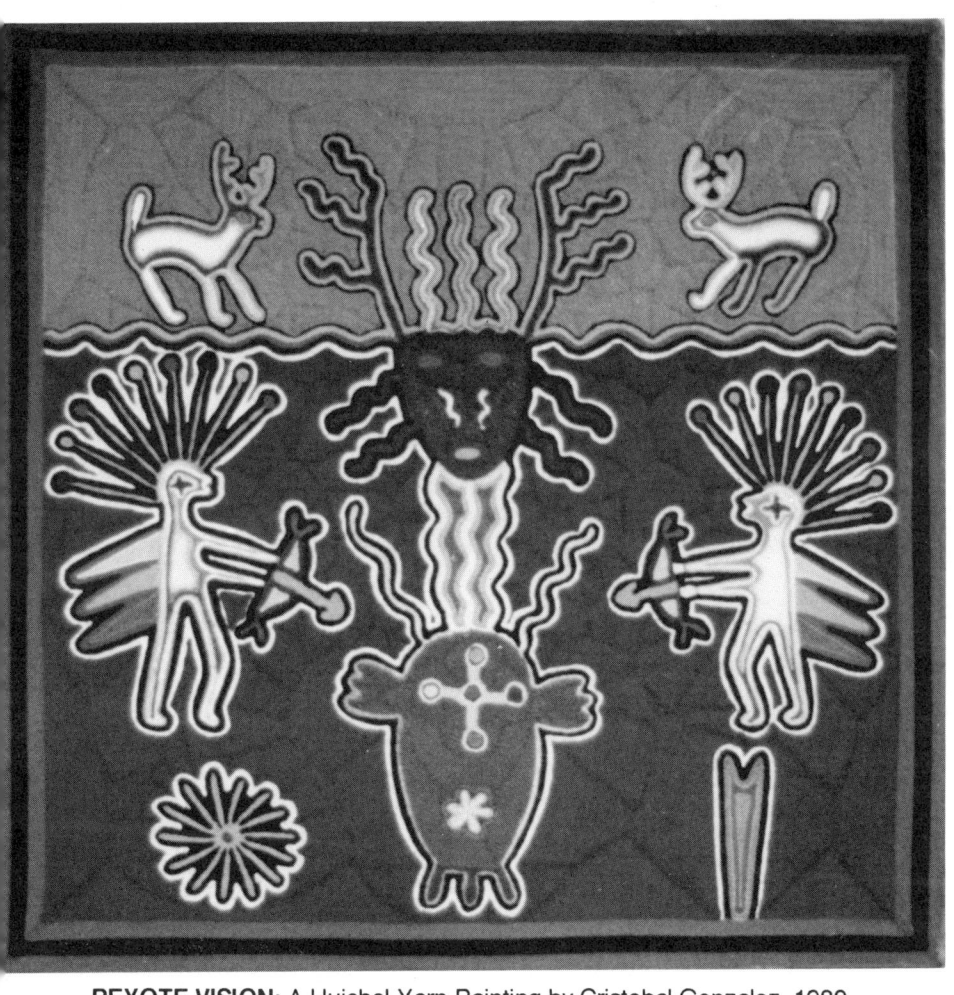

PEYOTE VISION: A Huichol Yarn Painting by Cristobal Gonzalez, 1980.

PART FIVE:
Scientific and Medical Reports

Scientific investigations of *Lophophora* reveal many therapeutic benefits and suggest that more studies would be appropriate. Peyote alkaloids are:

1) Antibiotic, showing a wide range of effectiveness against many strains of bacteria, particularly some types of penicillin-resistant bacteria.

2) Antiseptic, cleaning open cuts and wounds,and promoting a strong flexible scab that draws the skin together and seals it better than stitches.

3)Psychotherapeutic, curing alcoholism and drug addictions; relieving distress, acute depression (soul-loss), and other sorrows of life.

4) Spiritually Nourishing, providing food and medicine for the soul.

5) Non-toxic, no deaths or addictions have been attributed to peyote; it does not contain strychnine or anything else that is harmful.

5) A Home Remedy, safely used for centuries by native people to treat arthritis, rheumatism,pleurisy, common colds and flu, nerve spasms and paralysis, sciatica, blindness, hearing disorders, and to relieve the pain from broken bones and childbirth.

A remarkable study of the *"Effects of Peyote on Human Chromosomes"* by David Dorrance, MD (***Journal of the American Medical Association***, 1975—Vol.234, No. 3, Oct.) concluded that "...no significant chromosomal aberrations were apparent among the peyote—and non-peyote—using Huichol Indians." This study is important, because it should lay to rest the widespread rumor that peyote use somehow damages chromosomes.

—Guy Mount, Editor

There's A Big Difference
Between Peyote and A Pill

Lophophora williamsii represents a veritable factory of alkaloids. More that thirty alkaloids and their amine derivatives—have been isolated from the plant. Although most, if not all, of them are in some way or other biodynamically active, their effects are not well understood...The phenyl-etylamine mescaline is the vision-inducing alkaloid...Other alkaloids are undoubtably responsible for the tactile, auditory and occasionally other hallucinations of the peyote intoxication.

There are very real differences between peyote intoxication and mescaline intoxication. Among aboriginal users, it is the fresh or dried heads of the cactus, with its total alkaloid content, that is ingested; mescaline...produces the effects of but one of the alkaloids, without the physiological interaction of the others that are present in the crude plant material.

(Dried peyote buttons) are well-nigh indestructible, can be shipped long distances and store indefinitely.

—Richard E. Schultes
Director of the Botanical Museum
Harvard University

FLESH OF THE GODS, "An Overview of Hallucinogens in the Western Hemisphere:" Schultes, 1972.

Antibotic Activity
Of An Extract Of Peyote

The use of peyote in religious rites by many Indian tribes is common knowledge. In addition, curative properties for such varied ailments as toothache, pain in childbirth, fever, breast pain, skin diseases, rheumatism, diabetes, colds, and blindness, among other things, have been claimed for this plant by the same peoples...The *U.S. DISPENSATORY* lists peyote under the name *Anhalonium* and indicates its use to some extent in various forms for neurasthsenia and hysteria and also in cases of asthma...

Extracts of whole peyote plants were prepared in various solvents and screened for antimicrobial activity...and showed positive microbial inhibition...the principle antibiotic substance was given the name *Peyocactin.*

TABLE 1

Results of Antimicrobial Assay of Peyocactin

Organism	Activity of* Peyocactin	Organism	Activity of* Peyocactin
Agrobacterium tumefaciens	+ +	Proctus vulgaris	0
Bacillus cereus	+ +	Pseudomonas acruginosa	0
B. subtilis (USDA 220(	+ + +	Salmonella pullorum	0
Diplococcus pneumoniae	0	S. typhimurium	0
Escherichia coli (ATCC 6477)	+ + +	Sarcina lutea (USDA 1001(	+ + + +
Klebsiella pneumoniae	0	Shigella flexneri	+ +
Micrococcus flavus	+ + +	Staphylococcus aureus (USDA 209)	+ + +
M. rubens	+ + +	S. epidermitis	+ + +
Mycobacterium phlei	+ +	Streptococcus pyogenes	+ + + +
Neisseria catarrhalis	+ + +	S. salivaris	+ + +
Phytomonas campestris	+ + +	Candida Albicans	+

*   0 — no activity noted
     + — zone of inhibition only under Oxford cup
   + + — idem. 8 to 10 mm diameter
  + + + — idem. 11 to 15 mm diameter
 + + + + — idem. larger than 15 mm diameter

Swiss-Webster white mice were used for preliminary animal toxicity tests and protection studies to indicate the degree of inhibitory action of peotcactin against fatal staphyloccal infection. In every case the protected animals survived while those in the control group succumbed within 60 hours after infection with *S. aureus...*

Summary: A water-soluble crystalline substance separated from an ethanol extract of *Lophophora williamsii...* exhibited antibiotic activity against a wide spectrum of bacteria and a species of the imperfect fungi...Of particular interest was its inhibitory action against 18 strains of penicillin-resistant *Staphylococcus aureus*.

—David L. Walkington
Department of Bacteriology
University of Arizona

ECONOMIC BOTANY: Walkington, 1960.

Apparent Safety Of Peyote

Several states have passed laws against possession and use of peyote. However, very little evidence has been reported on this subject...My familiarity with the Native American Church has resulted from the day-to-day work of the mental health program on the Navajo area of the Indian Health Service working with the 125,000 Navajo Indians, the largest tribe in the United States...We provide consultation to many community organizations, including the Native American Church. As a result, we seem to have good success in case finding, and in general there is little reluctance to refer cases to us. Nevertheless, we have seen almost no acute or chronic emotional disturbance arising from peyote use.

For a period of four years we have followed up every report of psychotic or other psychiatric episodes said to have arisen from peyote use. There have been about 40 to 50 such reports, most of which were hearsay that could never be traced to a particular case. Some have been based on a physician's belief that Navajo people use peyote and that if a particular person became disturbed it must have been for this reason. There has been one relatively clear-cut case of acute psychosis and four cases that are difficult to interpret. (The "acute psychosis" occurred when a Navajo man attended a peyote meeting after drinking alcohol-Ed.) Assuming that all five of our cases represent true reactions to peyote and that we hear about half of the cases occurring,the resulting-probably over-estimated-rate would be approximately one bad reaction per 70,000 ingestions...This rate is much lower than others that have been reported for the use of hallucinogenic agents.

We have seen many patients come through difficult crises with the help of this religion. The Peyotists themselves are proud in particular of the help the church has been to Indian people who have drinking problems. In fact, Levy and Kunitz (1970) report a greater success rate for the Peyotists than for any other agency working with alcoholics in one part of the Navajo reservation.

—Dr. Robert Bergman, Chief
U.S. Public Health Service
Navajo Reservation, Arizona

❂

Discussion: I concur in all that Dr. Robert Bergman has said. I see the legal persecution that keeps cropping up as typical of the reactionary regression of the day...Peyote is not harmful to these people; it is beneficial, comforting, inspiring, and appears to be spiritually nourishing. It is a better antidote to alcohol than anything the missionaries, the white man, the American Medical Association, and the public health services have come up with. It is understandable that these organizations should be a bit envious of the success of this...natural native remedy.

—Dr. Karl A. Menninger
Topeka, Kansas

AMERICAN JOURNAL OF PSYCHIATRY: Bergman, 1971.

A Medical Report

While the main use of peyote among Indians has been ritualistic, it has also been used for healing purposes by Indians and whites. South Texas Mexicans used a decoction of the peyote "bulb" as a drink in fevers and as a lotion for the feet and head. It was used by the Indians as a pain killer, and it is reported that U.S. Army surgeons used it for the same purpose. Tribes of northern Mexico and southern Arizona chewed the root for application as a poultice to fractures, larger open wounds, and snakebite. It was supposed to have a beneficial effect on rheumatism and paralysis among the Kansas Potawatomis. Psycho-therapeutic effects have been attributed to it...

About the last decade of the previous century, clinical investigators were moved to examine the properties of peyote observing its use among Oklahoma Indians. True (1901) remarked that "hospital tests showed that the alkaloidal principle contained in the cactus furnishes a valuable remedy for certain troubles of the nervous system." Kluver (1928) believed that peyote offered a valuable instrument for clinical research in ophthalmology (a field of medicine concerned with structure, functions, and diseases of the eye) and psychiatry. *Anhalonium* is the pharmaceutical name of the drug, containing several alkaloids including mescaline, which is derived from this plant...

The most spectacular surgery performed in Pre-Columbian America was trephination (skull surgery), of which the most abundant evidence has been found in Peru, though trephined skulls have been found in several parts of the United States and Canada...in the operation Indians of the Andes employed several anesthetic drugs, including cocaine and peyote...in accordance with the surgical principle of fracture decompression, though perhaps with a view to releasing evil spirits.

—Virgil J .Vogel

AMERICAN INDIAN MEDICINE: Vogel, 1970.

Better Than Stitches

I taught at Lincoln Continuation High School for three years. Lincoln served young men and women who had been kicked out, dropped out, or otherwise found too far out for regular high school. The students were a good mix of pregnant teenagers, black and chicano street gangs, dopers, surfers, a few extraordinarily intelligent poets, artists, writers and thinkers, one or two prostitutes, several dealers, and other all-round good people, including an urban Navajo boy named John. He was in my basic reading class. One night John's mother Ann called me at home near midnight. She was asking for "Help, please, Mr. Mount! Would you talk to John? He needs stitches and won't go to the hospital. They cut his head.."

Ann was a trained nurse, so she knew about "stitches." I reluctantly agreed to talk John into going to a hospital, but he strongly declined the opportunity when we spoke.

"I'm afraid of a police report," he said. "Those other guys may come after me for saying anything. They hit me in the head with a 2X4, but I got them pretty good too." I asked to talk with Ann again, and volunteered to try "doctoring" John at my home with herbs.

"What kind of herbs?" Ann asked shyly.

"The kind your Navajo relatives use-Peyote," I said.

"We'll be right up, Mr. Mount," Ann replied. Then she drove fifty miles from Riverside to my house in the mountains. John's wound was terrible. His scalp was center-cut down the middle, down to the bone. The open wound was gray, pus-filled and street dirty, and slowly pumping blood. I gave John a button to eat and pray with, while I squeezed fresh peyote juices into the open cut. The bleeding stopped right away. The color turned from gray to pink. And within an hour John was sitting up straight, singing a song. We washed his hair and kept the wound full of juice. By dawn, Ann said the scalp scab looked better than stitches.

—Guy Mount, Teacher

Folk Medicine

Peyote is exhibited prominently today in the herb stalls of the Terron market...it is a versatile popular remedy, used internally and/or externally in the treatment of fever, shoulder pain, menstrual hemorrhage, vaginal discharge and rheumatism.

[The following quotations are remedies used by medicine men and women living in the Laguna district of Northern Mexico-Ed.]

488. Fever may be cured with peyote. It is ground on the metate; water is added and the preparation is strained. It is drunk sweetened with sugar. This is to cure all kinds of fever. Formerly it was used a great deal...

489. Peyote is very useful when one has pain in the shoulders...The peyote button is skinned and the flesh is roasted and then rubbed on the shoulder.

490. To stop menstrual hemorrhage, a bit of peyote is boiled with romero and pecan shell. With the water a vaginal douche is given, and a little of the tea is drunk. This treatment takes place, morning and night, for nine days.

491. I know very little of herbal remedies. The spirits give me my prescriptions. For example, they have told me that peyote is good for a pain in the shoulder and for an internal illness of women which results in a yellow discharge. This is cured with vaginal douches of peyote. A small piece is cooked—very small, for the medicine is

strong. First one heats the water. When it is boiling, one drops in a piece of peyote and covers the vessel, removing it from the fire. The douche is of a temperature desired (by the patient). It is given every other day (until she recovers).

492. For rheumatism or "tired" legs, (dry) peyote is pounded and added to alcohol. It is left to stand—one day is sufficient—and then the affected part is rubbed (with the liquid). One also takes a bit of peyote orally. A little water is heated—about one and a half cups. In it is dropped a small piece of peyote. The tea is drunk twice a day, in the morning before breakfast and at night; the treatment is repeated for nine or fifteen days. The remedy is the same for rheumatism and for "tired" legs.

—Isabel Kelly

FOLK PRACTICES IN NORTH MEXICO: Kelly, 1955. University of Texas Press, Austin TX.

Home Remedy

Recommended for complaints such as gum infections, sore throat, aching joints, muscle and nerve pain, loss of soul and physical strength:

Remove the white hairlike tufts from each button and any dry bark or soil. The medicine is most effective eaten fresh or dried. The organic juices, or undiluted peyote extract, can be applied to open cuts and wounds for antiseptic healing. The scab formed by peyote alkaloids is flexible and strong; it actually pulls the skin together like stitches, and stops bleeding.

Peyote extract or tea is made by placing one or more clean buttons in a pint of water. Bring them to a boil and reduce heat to simmer for an hour. The yellow-brown tea can be diluted with more water for a milder effect. Always drink peyote tea, or eat it, on an empty stomach and add prayer. It has a strong medicinal taste,"bitter" to some. "Sweet" to us. The vomiting associated with peyote use has more to do with what's in your mind and stomach than with anything in the medicine.

Peyote tea is also enjoyable when you are feeling healthy and can make almost any activity of the heart more delightful. One may feel especially blessed while working in a garden, playing music, making love, building a house, or creating artwork and crafts. Peyote is a tonic and stimulant.

One dried peyote button, the size of a quarter, has approximately 50 mg. of alkaloids. Perhaps 400-500 mg. of these combined alkaloids (mescaline alone is not the same as organic peyote) are required for a visionary experience, that is: seven or eight buttons. So called "organic mescaline" is usually LSD mixed with speed. The real medicine looks like a plant, not a pill.

WARNING: A peyote lesson can be as gentle as a baby, or as harsh as your lack of respect.

—Guy Mount, Editor

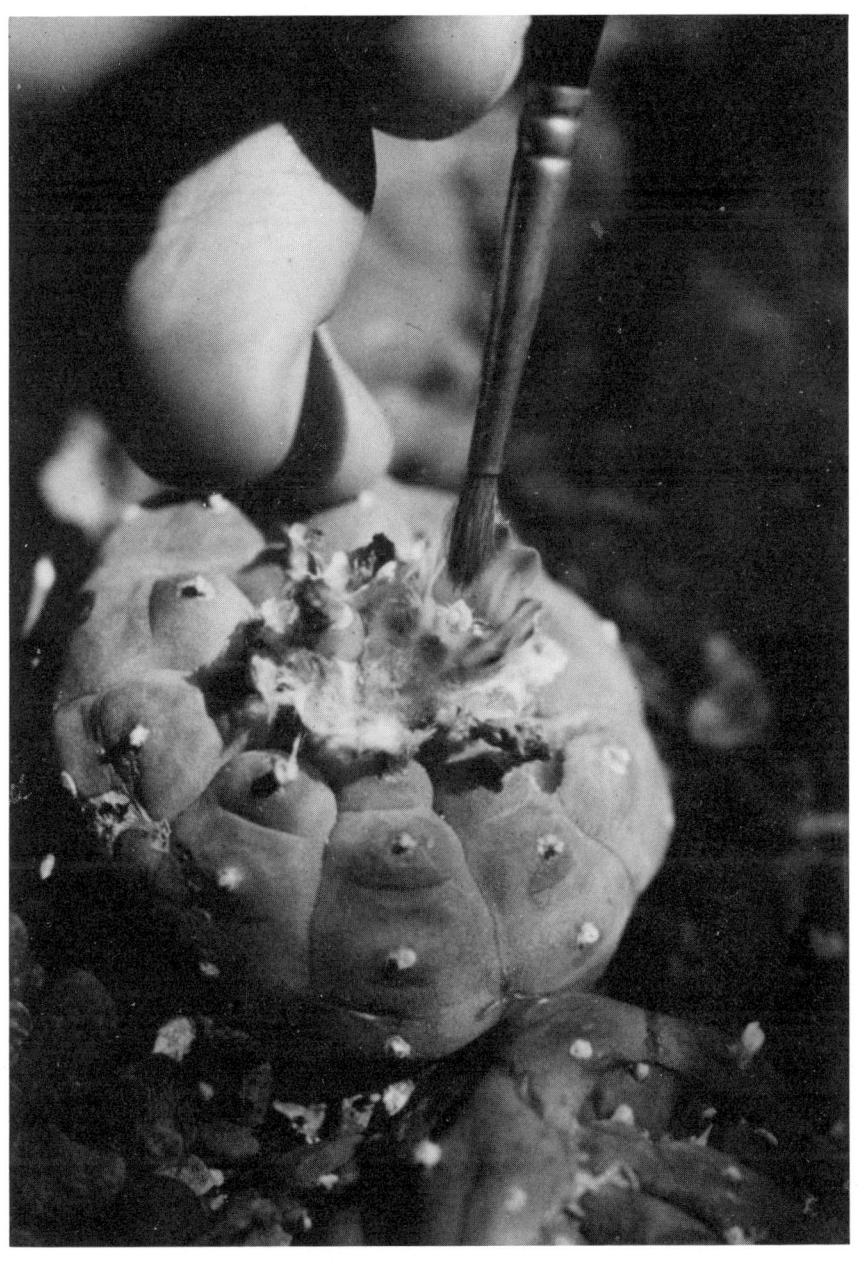

POLLINATION OF PEYOTE: Courtesy of Larry Noggle.

PART SIX:
Ecology and Cultivation of Peyote

Should the present laws against peyote use be changed, it is likely the demand for the medicine would increase beyond the natural supply. Therefore I have included some guidelines for the cultvation of *Lophophora* to help prevent extinction from over-harvesting.

Peyote was grown in commercial green houses legally prior to legislation passed during the Nixon administration, and shipped to consumers throughout the United States. It is still cultivated by individual collectors of cacti, and by local chapters of Native American and other peyote churches. My own experiments with the cultivation of seeds and cuttings confirm that *Lophophora* will grow vigorously, almost anywhere, providing that it is protected from cold damp weather, and too much direct sunlight. Temperatures in excess of 80 degrees will stimulate the growth and flowering of cuttings. All it needs is love and limestone soil.

—Guy Mount, Editor

Ecology of Peyote

General Characteristics of *Lophophora* Populations: Peyote is not a rare cactus and in many localities is quite abundant, often forming clumps under most sizable shrubs. Caeposite individuals or even large clones are common, although single headed plants are present in each locality as well. Injury or harvesting by man induces the formation of many stems from a single rootstock. Single clones more than 1.5 meters across have been observed in San Luis Potosi, for example.

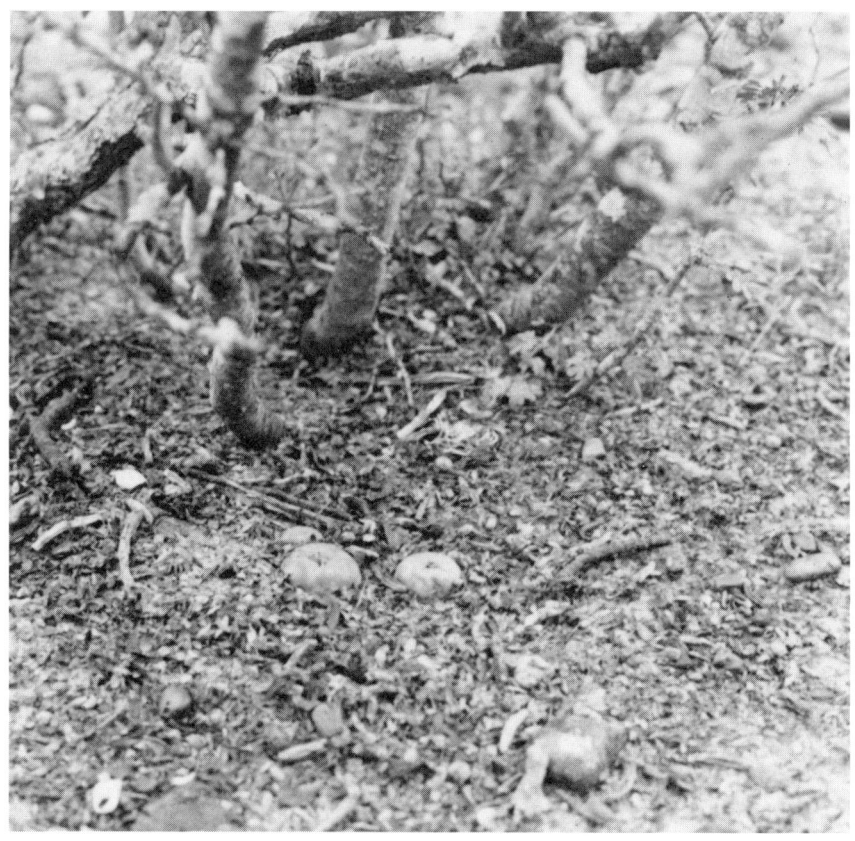

NATIVE MEDICINE by Guy Mount

Although it is not uncommon to encounter it in full sunlight, *Lophophora* tends to grow under associated shrubs such as *Larrea* and *Prosopis* or in the partial shade of plants such as *Agave.*

Lophophora has been observed growing in silty limestone flood plains or wedged between rocks on nearly vertical limestone cliffs, but it occurs most frequently on low limestone hills and plains composed of broken and flaky limestone.

Reproduction is primarily sexual, and often young plants can be found growing in or around mature ones. Asexual reproduction can also occur by the formation of new stems from old. These can become detached (by man, animals, wind, water, etc.) and sometimes they will root during the rainy season.

The age and size of the plant are two factors that apparently determine the number of ribs on plants of the northern population. Young plants normally have five, but mature individuals may have 5-14 or occasionally none at all. This range of rib variation can occur within the same clump, so apparently it is a response to various factors. *Lophophora,* especially the large northern population, exhibits a wide range of environmental morphological variations...

"Lophophora" is derived from two Greek words meaning "I bear crest," referring to the "crests" of trichomes borne on each tubercle. Common names are peyote, piote, piotl, challote, mescal, rais diabolica, dry whiskey, dumpling cactus, and tuna de tierra. There are also numerous names in the Indian languages.

—Edward F. Anderson

BRITTONIA MAGAZINE, "The Biogeography, Ecology, and Taxonomy of Lophophora (Cactacea). " Anderson, 1969.

Cultivation of *Lophophora*

Peyote has been cultivated for centuries. It was one of many medicinal herbs found in the famous Aztec Gardens of Montezuma, and it was grown commercially in the United States until fairly recently. The ease with which peyote can be transplanted or sprouted from seeds is the major reason why the plant has not become ecologically extinct.

Lophophora species can be cultivated from seeds or cuttings like most cacti. The only special requirement is a limestone-based soil mixture. Peyote seeds germinate quickly (3 to 7 days), but require two years or more to mature and flower. Some plants live to be a hundred and generate many children from the parent rootstock. These cuttings—carefully removed—should be kept absolutely dry and shaded. Never freeze or refrigerate peyote. It retains full medicinal potency indefinitely in the dried state and the potential for regrowth when potted. Cool, damp conditions will rot the plant and its seeds, as well as destroy the alkaloid content. Peyote tolerates most anything except freezing temperatures and excessive moisture.

Peyote seeds are located inside tiny seedpods (berries)which form beneath the flowers after fertilization. The seedpods are ordinarily hidden and protected by the silky white tufts at the center of a button. By carefully removing the tufts with a fingernail it is possible to find loose seeds and pods. Sometimes 25 to 30 small black or red seeds, the size of a pinhead, are found in a single seedpod. I have found more than a hundred seeds in one button, containing four seedpods. These should be kept dry and out of the light until planted.

The key to successful cultivation of seeds and cuttings is a limestone soil mixture. The following information may prove helpful in getting the right mix:

1) Peyote was grown commercially in New Mexico. One grower I visited recommends pure gypsum. He simply pulverizes a piece of ordinary gypsum board, the type used in house construction called "dry wall" and adds this powder to coarse sand. I saw one clone of peyote with 30 individual buttons that had branched off from the roots of an older plant. This grandparent plant and family were growing in an enamel washpan that contained about four inches of sandy gypsum. Holes were punched in the bottom of the pan for good drainage. His peyote seedlings were growing in clay pots containing gypsum. These sprouts were an inch in diameter after six months' growth. Of course, his greenhouse was situated in a desert environment south of Albuquerque along the Rio Grande, where the intense heat stimulates maximum growth. His plants were shaded and dry.

2) My own soil mixture came from the limestone hills along the Rio Grande in southern Texas. It is a blend of crushed limestone, coarse sand and desert topsoil. It includes rotted leaves and rabbit manure. It has excellent drainage, which prevents rot—the main enemy of cacti plants.

3) Cuttings will grow in commercial potting soil for cacti in general, which can be obtained from any gardening center. I would add gypsum, and use organic fertilizer once roots had formed and new growth was obvious. Dolomite lime, available commercially, is a good substitute for gypsum.

4) A chemical analysis (Anderson, 1969) of the soil found where peyote grows naturally indicates:

"All soils tested were limestone in origin, with a basic PH (7.9-8.3). These soils can also be characterized as having more than 150 ppm Ca, at least 6ppm Mg., strong carbonates, and no more than trace amounts of NH3. The soils tested negatively for Ge, Cl, SO4, Mn , and Al. Four sites tested positively for NO3 and six showed NO3 to be present. Phosphorous and potassium varied somewhat throughout the range, no more than 3ppm P were present at any site. Two localities...showed considerable K, whereas the other sites showed either trace amounts or none at all. Soil tests from the southernmost locality in Queretaro were not different from those of more northern soils."

Once a soil mixture has been prepared, peyote seeds can be germinated in ordinary clay pots. Sprinkle seeds an inch apart and bury slightly beneath the surface. Water the pot from below with rainwater, if possible, or other pure water. Cover the pot with a opaque plastic lid or pane of glass. Prop the cover open with a toothpick to admit some air, but maintain humidity necessary for proper germination. Lack of ventilation will cause molds and bacteria to multiply on the surface of the soil mixture, and later attack the plants at soil level. Too much air and the seeds will not germinate because moisture will not soak through the tough seedcoat. Place the pot in a hot shady spot outdoors, or in a heated closet with light.

Direct sunshine will burn tender sprouts and older potted plants as well. Keep them shaded and remove the cover when a majority of seeds have sprouted, which should be within one week. Water as often as the soil dries out, but keep all plants on the dry side.

With all cacti, too much water is worse than none at all. Desert plants live several years without water, and so do potted cacti. Gradually expose seedlings and new transplants to full daylight, but not direct sunlight until they are well established. Discontinue watering of all peyote plants during the late fall and keep them dry throughout winter. If the plants are kept in a heated room, they may be watered on occasion to prevent undue shriveling.

Peyote buttons which have a sizable rootstock can be transplanted as cuttings. The wound can be treated with sulfur powder or charcoal dust, then allowed to form a dry callous. When the wound is completely healed, the plant can be potted in a limestone soil mixture. It should be kept warm, dry and shaded. Cuttings make new roots best during the springtime when night temperatures remain above 70 degrees. The yearly cycle and warmth of spring is essential for stimulating new growth. Normally, peyote lies dormant for a brief period each year. When new growth and plumpness indicate that roots have formed, water sparingly with rabbit manure tea.

Good luck and many blessings.

—Guy Mount, Editor

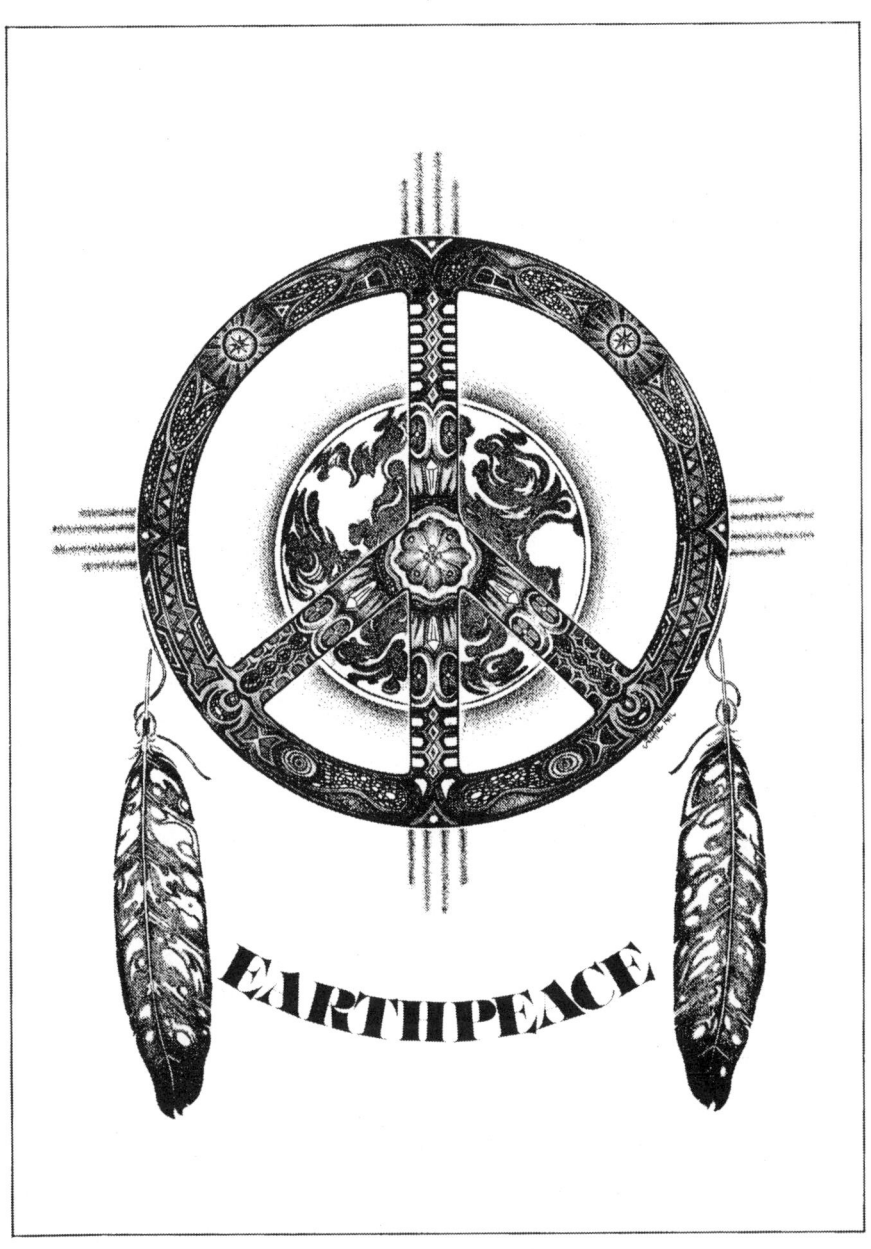

A Color Greeting Card
by Jeffree' Hall
Copyright © by SPIRIT GRAPHICS
Box 1656, Jacksonville, OR 97530

PART SEVEN:
Peyote And The Law

We need spiritual freedom in America. The peyote religion has been a lifeline from the past for native people. I believe it can be a lifeline to the future for many others. But the truth is the Peyote Religion has been suppressed by laws which discriminate against followers according to their race, and by ideas which discredit the Good Medicine by classifying it as a dangerous drug.

In California, for example, the rights of Native Americans seem protected because of a favorable decision by the California Supreme Court in the 1964 "Woody Case." However the rights of non-Indian peyotists are ambiguous at best since their use of peyote is a felony under state law despite the fact that peyote proves to be spiritually nourishing and medically beneficial regardless of ethnic ancestry, and despite the alleged constitutional right to religious freedom for all Americans.

Three states have exempted peyote from "controlled substance" prohibitions, and do permit the "bona-fide" sacramental use of peyote by non-Indians who are members of an established church: these are New York, Arizona and New Mexico. The Federal District Court of New York decided in 1979 that "the use of peyote for sacramental purposes...is not to be restricted solely to the Native American Church." Thus a precedent has been clearly established, and under Arizona laws the Peyote Way Church of God was licensed as perhaps the first all-race organization with appropriate authority. A recent decision by the Supreme Court of the United States (1990) makes it clear that we do not have a constitutional right to use any controlled substance as a religious sacrament. Instead, each state has the right to pass laws which honor the peyote religion, or continue to suppress it. Apparently the First Amendment only applies to established religions.

The same Peyote Way Church which is legal in Arizona has encountered difficulties in Texas, where church members were arrested for harvesting medicine. Charges were dismissed, but the Church filed a countersuit against Texas for discrimination, noting that members of the Native American Church were permitted to harvest and purchase peyote from local licensed dealers. This would seem to be a case of obvious racial and religious discrimination on the part of Texas, but in a decision that makes a mockery of American history, the Fifth Circuit Court declared that "Indian Nations were sovereign entities" with special rights to all of the peyote in the United States. Therefore members of the Peyote Way Church, with membership open to all people regardless of ethnic ancestry, could not pick or purchase peyote in Texas. I would think the previously unrecognized "Indian Nations" could now use the language of this decision to sue Texas for the return of their sovereign land and other natural resources. The American legislative and judicial system conveniently recognizes Sovereign Indian Nations only when that point of view perpetuates the empire.

If the state of Texas really cared about Indian rights, or preventing the depletion of the natural peyote gardens by non-Indian peyotists, it would encourage commercial cultivation of peyote and develop a peyote nature preserve in Starr County, which had a perpetual harvest plan for providing medicine to the Native American Church. This would put many south Texas ranchers back in business, after years of recession-economics. And perhaps the Native American Church might be more supportive of non-Indian rights, if the increasingly diminishing natural supply of peyote were not threatened by a growing demand.

—Guy Mount, Editor

The Woody Case

The *Woody et al.* case was appealed to the California Supreme Court and an opinion favorable to peyotism freed Jack Woody, Leon Anderson, and Dan Dee Nez. The opinion delivered on August 24, 1964, was written by Justice J. Tobriner and was concurred in by five or six other justices. Justice Tobriner wrote:

> On the other hand, the right to free religious expression embodies a precious heritage of our history. In a mass society, which presses at every point toward conformity, the protection of self-expression, however unique, of the individual and the group becomes ever more important. The varying currents of the subcultures that flow into the mainstream of our national life give depth and beauty. We preserve a greater value than an ancient tradition when we protect the rights of the Indians who honestly practiced an old religion in using peyote one night at a meeting in a desert hogan near Needles, CA."

Since the California law remained unchanged in spite of the California Supreme Court ruling, Navaho Indians and others discovered transporting peyote in California are at times arrested and held until the local district attorney learns of the *Woody et al.* case and of the exemption given by the court when peyote is used in a bona fide religious ceremony.

—Omer C. Stewart

PEYOTE RELIGION: A History by Omer C. Stewart, 1987.
University of Oklahoma Press: Norman, OK.

California Law

11352. Transportation, sale, giving away, etc. of designated controlled substances; punishment for peyote.

(a) Except as otherwise provided in this division, every person who transports, imports into this state, sells, furnishes, administers or gives away, or offers to transport, import into this state, sell, furnish, administer, or give away, or attempts to import into this state or transport (1) any controlled substance specified in subdivision (b) or (c) of Section 11054, or specified in subdivision (b) or (c) of Section 11055, or (2) any controlled substance classified in Schedule III, IV, or V which is a narcotic drug, unless upon the written prescription of a physician, dentist, podiatrists, or veterinarian licensed to practice in this state, shall be punished by imprisonment in the state prison for a period of five years to life and shall not be eligible for release upon completion of sentence or on parole or any other basis until he has been imprisoned for a period of not less that three years in the state prison.

(b) If such person has been previously convicted shall be charged in the indictment of information and, if found to be true by the jury upon a jury trial or by the court upon a court trial or if admitted by the person, he shall be imprisoned in the state prison for a period of 10 years to life and shall not be eligible for release upon completion of sentence or on parole or any other basis until he has been imprisoned for a period of not less than10 years in the state prison.

(c) If such person has been previously convicted two or more times of any offense described in subdivision (d), the previous convictions shall be charged in the indictment or information and, if found to be true by the jury upon a jury trial or by the court upon a court trial or if admitted by the person, he shall be imprisoned in the state prison for a period of 15 years to life and shall not be eligible for release upon completion of sentence or on parole or any other basis until he has been imprisoned for a period of not less than 15 years in the state prison.

11363. Planting, cultivating and harvesting; punishment for peyote.

(a) Every person who plants, cultivates, harvests, dries, or processes any plant of the genus *Lophophora,* also known as peyote, or any part thereof shall be punished by imprisonment in the county jail for a period of not more than one year or the state prison for a period of not more than 10 years.

(b) If such person has been previously convicted of any offense described in subdivision (c), the previous conviction shall be charged in the indictment or information and, if found to be true by the jury upon a jury trial or by the court upon a court trial or if admitted by the person, he shall be imprisoned in the state prison for a period of not less than two years or more than 20 years.

Federal Court Finding: New York D.C., 1979

17. Religious uses

Under this chapter, the use of peyote for sacramental purposes where peyote is regarded as a deity is not to be restricted solely to the Native American Church, a religious organization of American Indians, and thus exemption for peyote was equally available to plaintiff church if in fact it was a bona fide religious organization and would make use of peyote for sacramental purposes and regard the the drug as a deity. Native American Church of New York v. U.S. D.C.N.Y., 1979, 468 F. Supp. 1247 affirmed 633 F 2d 205.

Plaintiff church was not entitled to relief from provisions of this chapter for so-called psychedelic drugs, other than peyote, allegedly used as a sacrament or aid to worship. Id.

A Texas Decision

Judge Maloney of the Fifth Circuit Court ruled against the Peyote Way Church of God in Arizona on October 28, 1988 stating that:

1) There is a limited supply of the Holy Sacrament peyote, and all of it is needed for the Native American Church of North America.

2) The government is authorized to make laws to protect the public even if those laws infringe on the Church's religious rights, therefore the Federal and Texas State drug laws are legitimate.

3) Federal and Texas State laws are not racist, they're political. Native American Church members belong to a sovereign nation.

"The court therefore concludes that regardless of the sincerity of Peyote Way's members' beliefs in peyotism, the exemption provided the Native American Church cannot be expanded to include non-Native American Church use of peyote.

The Court further concludes that the overriding interest of Congress to control the use of narcotics and psychotropic drugs outweighs the interest of expanding an exemption that clearly was meant to be a grandfather clause, and not a full-scale exemption of religious peyote use.

Finding that Congress' intent to exempt the Native American Church is not meant to extend to other Churches which use peyote, the Court finds that Peyote Way's claims for violation of the free exercise clause and establishment clause of the First Amendment must fail."

—Judge Robert Maloney
U.S. District Court Judge

Courtesy of Rev. Anne L. Zapf, President
Peyote Way Church Of God

U.S. Supreme Court Report

Employment Division
Department of Human Resources of Oregon, et al., Petitioners
v
Alfred L. Smith et al.

[No. 88-1213] 494 US 872, 108 L Ed 2nd 876, 110 S Ct 1595

Argued November 6, 1989. Decided April 17, 1990.

Decision: Oregon's prohibition of use of peyote in religious ceremony held not to violate free exercise of religion clause of Federal Constitution's First Amendment.

SUMMARY

Two drug rehabilitation counselors, both of whom were members of the Native American Church, were fired from their jobs with a private corporation in Oregon because they had ingested peyote, a hallucinogenic drug, for sacramental purposes at a ceremony of the Church. The counselors applied to the Employment Division of Oregon's Department of Human Resources for unemployment compensation, but the department's Employment Appeals Board ultimately denied their applications on the ground that the counselors had been discharged for misconduct connected with work. The Oregon Court of Appeals, reversing the boards's decisions, (1) held that the denial of benefits to persons who were discharged for engaging in a religious act constituted an unjustified burden on the right of free exercise of religion, and (2) remanded the cases to the board for further findings as to the religious nature of the counselors' acts (75 Or App 764, 707 P2d 1274, 709 P2d 246). The Supreme Court of Oregon, holding that such further findings were unnecessary and that the counselors were entitled to payment of unemployment benefits, affirmed both judgments as modified (301 Or 209, 221, 721 P2d 445, 451). On certiorari, the United States Supreme Court (1) noted that the Oregon Supreme Court had not decided whether the counselors' sacramental use of peyote was in fact proscribed by Oregon's controlled substance law, and that this issue was a matter of dispute between the parties, (2) determined that it would not be appropriate, given this uncertainty, for the United States Supreme Court to decide whether the practice was protected by the Federal Constitution, and accordingly (3) vacated the Oregon Supreme Court's judgment and remanded the case for further proceedings (485 US 660, 99 L Ed 2nd 753, 108 S Ct 1444). On remand, the Oregon Supreme Court held that (1) the

Oregon statute made no exception for the sacramental use of peyote, (2) the counselors' use of peyote thus fell within the prohibition of the statute, (3) the prohibition of the practice at issue was not valid under the free exercise clause of the Federal Constitution's First Amendment, and (4) the counselors could not be denied unemployment benefits for having engaged in that practice (307 Or 68, 763 P2d 146).

On certiorari, the United States Supreme Court reversed. In an opinion by Scalia, J., joined by Rehnquist, Ch. J., and White, Stevens and Kennedy, JJ., it was held that (1) the free exercise of religion clause permits a state to include religiously inspired use of peyote within the reach of the state's general criminal prohibition on use of that drug, where there is no contention that the state's drug law represents an attempt to regulate religious beliefs, the communication of religious beliefs, or the raising of one's children in those beliefs; (2) the free exercise of religion clause thus permitted Oregon to deny unemployment benefits to persons dismissed from their jobs because of such religiously inspired use; and (3) generally applicable, religion-neutral criminal laws that have the effect of burdening a particular religious practice need not be justified, under the free exercise of religion clause, by a compelling governmental interest.

O'Connor, J., concurred in the judgment and, in an opinion joined in part (as to points 1-3 below) by Brennan, Marshall, and Blackmun, JJ., expressed the view that (1) the question under the free exercise of religion clause was properly presented in the United States Supreme Court, (2) an individual's free exercise of religion is burdened by neutral laws of general applicability that make criminal the individual's religiously motivated conduct, (3) the First Amendment requires at least a case-by-case determination whether such a burden on specific individuals is constitutionally significant and whether the particular criminal interest asserted by the government is compelling, and (4) under such a test, (a) Oregon had a compelling interest in regulating peyote use by its citizens, (b) a selective exemption from the prohibition would unduly interfere with this interest, and therefore (c) the free exercise of religion clause did not require Oregon to accommodate the counselors conduct.

Blackmun, J., joined by Brennan and Marshall, JJ., dissenting, expressed the view that (1) a state statute that burdens the free exercise of religion may stand only if the law in general, and the state's refusal to allow a religious exemption in particular, are justified by a compelling interest that cannot be served by less restrictive means, (2) Oregon's interest in refusing to make an exception for the religious use of peyote was not sufficiently compelling to outweigh the counselors' right to the free exercise of their religion, and therefore (3) Oregon could not, consistent with the free exercise of religion clause, deny the counselors unemployment benefits.

A Real Commitment

Peyotism today echoes the longstanding problem of its opposition by the dominant population—the Spanish in Mexico and other Americans in the United States, government officials, Christian missionaries, educators, and U.S. senators and representatives. Legally, peyotists today have won their fight for religious freedom in the United States. Since 1978, with the passage of the American Indian Religious Freedom Act (42 USC I996, P.L./ 95-341), the practice of peyotism by American Indians is protected by law. This act orders all federal agencies to be aware of American Indian sacred sites, objects, plants, materials, etc.., and to protect them from destruction, if possible, and to make their use available to Indians. Peyotism is one of the several American Indian religions named as needing protection. But there is still the possibility of harassment of peyotists under the Drug Abuse Control Act of 1965, which includes peyote among prohibited narcotics, and many state laws which have similar restrictions. While a test in court will clear anyone of arrest for possession of peyote if it is shown that the peyote is for use in a ceremony of the NAC and that the possessor is a member of the NAC, the arrest and detainment can be discouraging. NAC members are learning to be careful not to carry peyote around with them, to carry identification of membership in some NAC congregation, and to know the law. While the efforts to enforce the Drug Control Act where it involves peyote may be an annoyance, most Peyotists are willing to conform to the law.

An unusual case of harassment under the Drug Control Act took place in Grand Forks, North Dakota, in October, 1984, when a white couple, Mr. and Mrs. John D. Warner, were arrested by the FBI for possessing peyote, a controlled drug. The two were members of the NAC of Tokio, North Dakota, and had been for a number of years, and Mrs. Warner was custodian of the supply of peyote for the Tokio congregation. The FBI had learned of the possession of peyote by the Warners from the president of the NAC of NA, Emerson Jackson (Navajo), so it was he who brought them to trial. Jackson said that they were not bona fide members of the NAC because they were not Indians. He maintained that in 1982 a motion had been passed by the NAC of NA to the effect that membership in that organization be limited to persons with one-quarter Indian blood, thereby excluding this white couple. A jury trial in Grand Forks Federal Court found the defendants innocent of breaking the law, since they were able to prove that although they were not Indians, nevertheless they were members in good standing of the local congregation of peyotists. The charges were dismissed.

This case not only illustrates harassment under the Drug Control Act, but it also brings up the legality of non-Indians as bona fide members of the NAC. From the beginning, attendance of non-Indians to peyote meetings has been a somewhat personal or tribal matter. For instance, very early in Oklahoma some Caddo refused to allow non-Indians to attend any of their meetings. But others, such as the Kiowa and Comanche, welcomed non-Indians, black or white, as long as they were seriously interested. With the formation of the NAC, the same attitude has generally prevailed, and the presence of non-Indians has been no problem. It was in the sixties when the hippie generation became interested in peyote and became a nuisance in the peyote gardens of Texas, bringing about the Texas law which forbids possession of peyote by persons not having one-quarter Indian blood and proof of membership in the NAC, that race became an issue in membership. Since then, if non-Indians wish to be allowed to possess peyote, they must show that their involvement in the peyote religion is genuine—that it is not just a recreational, frivolous, or passing interest but a real commitment. Then, as the case against the Warners shows, race is not an issue. Still, it is especially important for non-Indians to carry identification of membership in the NAC if they have occasion to carry peyote, and even so, non-Indians possessing peyote violate Texas law.

The ruling of the NAC of NA that only Indians should be enrolled in the Native American Church is new and is not shared by most peyotists. The NAC of NA does not speak for all peyotists, much as it would like to do so. All peyotists consider themselves members of the Native American Church, but most are not affiliated with the NAC of NA. Each congregation makes its own rules, just as each meeting is conducted by its own roadman.

—Omer C. Stewart

PEYOTE RELIGION: A HISTORY by Omer C. Stewart,1987.
University of Oklahoma Press: Norman, OK.

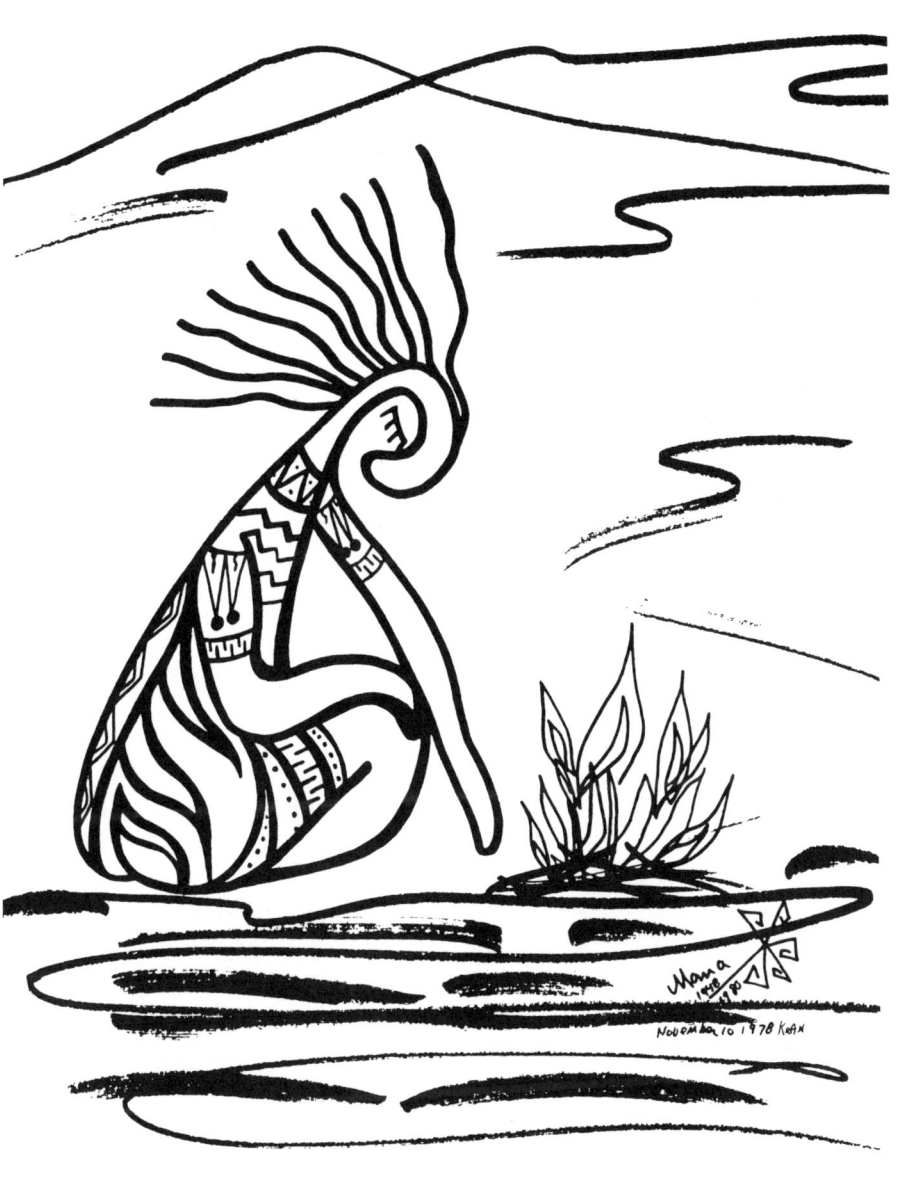

SPIRIT QUEST by Mana
Courtesy of The Peyote Way Church Of God.

PART EIGHT:
Conclusion and Testimonials

At this moment in American History, the practitioners of alternative herbal medicine and religion are the most persecuted and prosecuted members of society. Peyote itself is under attack from oil well development companies, dry land ranching techniques, and an ever increasing number of consumers. There is an immediate need to 1) pass laws in each state that protect the rights of all people, regardless of race or ethnic origin, to practice the peyote religion and pursue alternative healing strategies (which may employ herbs on the "controlled substances" list), and 2) protect peyote by developing nature preserves in south Texas and encouraging cultivation. The Peyote Religion and the herbal sacrament it depends on will soon be extinct unless something radical is done to establish environmental protection and decriminalize cultivation.

There is also a great need to provide educational curriculum that supports a peaceful transition from an abusive "War on Drugs" to a knowledgable use of herbal medicines. Our educational system presently teaches children that "drug use" is crazy and criminal. There is no distinction made between herbs and drugs, nor are any positive images of herbal medicines provided; so it's not surprising that American teenagers act crazy and commit crimes when they use herbs and drugs—that's what they've been taught to do!

Fortunately, the Native American Church and Native American philosophy in general provide us with the lessons we need to grow as individuals, and to improve the overall health of our society. Insofar as America learned from its native people, it has provided Light to the world through democracy, religious freedom and economic reciprocity. Therefore, I hope the Peyote Religion will grow substantially in the near future to include many new practitioners from all races, and legal Peyote Churches and greenhouses in all states. Our world needs this medicine, this lifeline to the future.

—Guy Mount, Editor

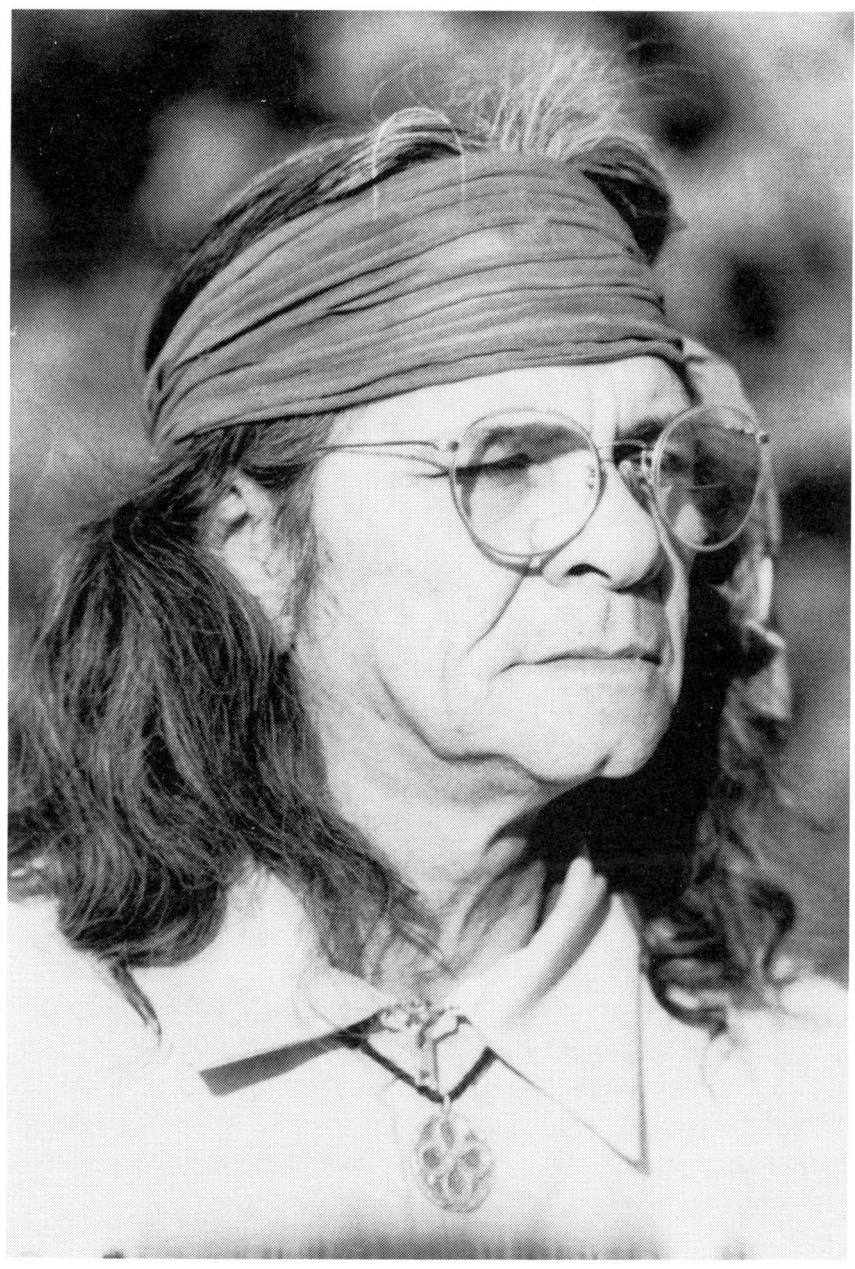

Reverend Immanuel P. Trujillo helped establish the all-race Peyote Way Church of God in Arizona.

The Peyote Way Church of God

My husband, Matthew, and I had been married one year when we first came to the 160 acres of holy land in the Aravaipa Valley, now known as The Peyote Way Church of God. We had experienced an unusual honeymoon, traveling through Mexico and Central America in search of spiritual direction. We met a loving and special man who helped us realize that the only path that would bring us lasting satisfaction was a spiritual one. He convinced us that we needn't smoke cigarettes, drink alcohol, or eat animal flesh.

When we returned to the United States we decided to settle in the Southwest. We considered a community in New Mexico, but met a man who had been to the Church of Holy Light, as it was then known, and decided to go see it for ourselves. When we arrived we saw—as our friend had said—that there were trees full of apples, and more fruit rotting on the ground. The land was beautiful and wild, but we could see the place needed attention.

Our friend took us inside the ranch-style house to a small room where we met Rev. Immanuel Trujillo, who was sitting at a table scraping clay cups. Matthew knelt before him so they could see eye to eye (there were no other chairs, except the ones occupied by two apprentices who were also busily scraping clay pots). My husband, Matthew, told Immanuel he was "looking for a boat to row."

I am sure Reverend Trujillo had heard such statements many times, because he smiled and began discussing a place called "Healing Waters" in Eden, Arizona. Shortly afterwards, Immanuel took us to Healing Waters, but we knew we wanted a different vocation with heart. We were relieved when Immanuel returned and took us back to the Church of Holy Light.

We were introduced to the holy sacrament peyote and to the making of earthenware pottery over the next several months. As our experiences with the medicine and this holy land grew, we came to feel strongly that we had found our home.

One day, Reverend Trujillo introduced us to the idea of declaring our religious belief in peyote as a sacrament. We composed a "Declaration of Intent" to steward and distribute the holy sacrament peyote, and took a large and beautiful peyote plant to the office of Graham County Superior Court Judge Ruskin Lines. We showed him the holy plant and asked if we would be going to jail? He smiled and said, "No."

Then the Judge asked Reverend Trujillo, who is 50% Apache, about the traditional Teepee Ceremony of the Native American Church. We spoke with the Judge for several minutes and left the holy peyote with him. The Judge wanted to show the plant to the Sheriff and Police Departments. Judge Lines returned the healthy smiling plant to us one month later.

During that time we recorded our Declaration of Intent with the Graham County Recorder's Office. The Peyote Way Church of God was incorporated in Arizona May 11, 1979.

The Church has been a place of prayer, meditation and miracles for us, as well as our many annual visitors and Spirit Walk communicants, including the miracle of my first pregnancy five years after Matthew's vasectomy. We now have two miraculous home birth children: a daughter, Joy, and son, Joseph.

Though we are all on vows of poverty our lives are spiritually rich, thanks to the holy sacrament peyote. The experience of God is beyond description, beyond words, and so that is why I dwell on the message rather than the experience. We do not discuss our personal experiences so much, because we want each communicant (who takes a Spirit Walk) to experience the holy sacrament without a lot of preconceptions. Each individual can have their own personal testimony of God through the sacrament of peyote.

I believe the "hand of God" led us to the holy sacrament peyote, and it is through the holy sacrament that we experience God. Peyote has guided and shaped my life and the life of my family. Our dietary guidelines, our ideas about childbirth, homeschooling, environmental pollution, disease, drugs and death have all come through the holy sacrament peyote. Our lifestyle of making pottery to sustain the Church, and the stamina to face the United States Government in its many forms of harassment upon us are Grace from God, received perhaps because we are obedient to the promptings received in revelation through the holy sacrament peyote.

We offer our prayers to God in the Spirit Walk, Fast Day Tea, and in remembrance when, at times, we may place a button in our cheek as we go about our daily meditations. It is on these occasions that I glimpse, or otherwise experience the fullness of my Lord.

Yours in "Its" service, remembering that God is infinite, endless and eternal—neither male, nor female.

—Reverend Anne L. Zapf, President

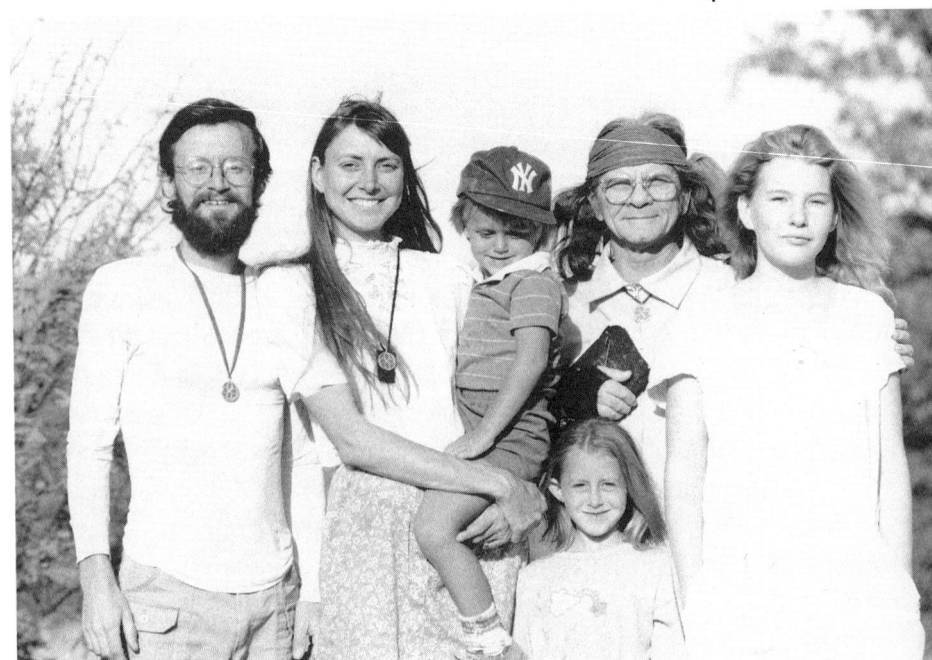

Rabbi Matthew S. Kent, Rev. Anne L. Zaph and their children with **Rev. Immanuel Trujillo** and his granddaughter, 1988.

Through The Lens Of Perception

"For now we see through a glass, darkly; but then face to face: now I know in part; but then shall I know even as also I am known." —I Corinthians

Nearly thirty years ago, I spent a summer in Mexico, much of it in a small village two hours by bus up the coast from Acapulco. As far as I know, the village had no name but was referred to as "the turnaround" (in Spanish, of course) because it was here that the third-class bus turned around and headed back over the mountain to Acapulco. I had gone there on the recommendation of a friend to escape the modern hotels and the tourist crowd. But I was not entirely prepared for the primitive conditions I met, or for a certain adventure that came to me. Instead of a modern hotel room, I found myself sleeping on a cot, covered only by a light sheet, just one of seven other rugged souls who had chosen this thatched roof dormitory over the more elegant accommodations available two hours south.

We always arose at sunrise, helped fold the cots, then stashed them away in one corner of the room. That done, we sat around and sipped coffee from crude, terra-cotta cups as we waited for breakfast to be served by the proprietor and his wife. Eating and sleeping under these conditions, created a bond between strangers, in spite of the language barriers. I knew enough Spanish to ask for basic life essentials, and the others, mostly Mexican students from the City, knew enough English to make small-talk.

One afternoon I met a man on the beach who said he was a tourist guide. He offered to take me up to the top of the mountain—I do not think I ever heard the name of it—where he promised to show me the most spectacular view imaginable. The fee for this jaunt was reasonable, and having nothing better to do I agreed to go with him.

The man's name was "Sen", and he was a wiry but strong looking little man who appeared to be in his early sixties. He wore only faded khaki pants and a red T-shirt with a flying hawk emblazoned across the chest. Underneath the bird, written in Spanish, was the name of a local beer. Sen was dark-skinned and had long black hair that reached nearly to his shoulders. His face had sharp Indian features, and when he smiled he revealed two front teeth capped in gold.

Just after noon, Sen packed a small knapsack with staples that he purchased from a *groceria* a short ways from our camp. Then we set out on foot in the most casual way imaginable. He pointed to the mountain peak where we were going. It looked to me to be miles and miles away. He assured me, however, that it was a much shorter distance than it looked, and I was not to worry.

We traveled on foot for most of the afternoon, taking what he called "El Sombre"—the shaded trail on the eastern slopes of the mountain, which protected us from the torturous rays of the afternoon sun. The trail was difficult, very steep at times, and not well maintained. I failed to keep track of the time, but we must have traveled for at least four hours before we stopped.

Finally Sen announced that we had arrived at our destination, and he led me to the mouth of a large cave, where we sat down to rest. I would guess that the cave was approximately two thousand feet above the sea. Less than a mile to the west, and seemingly straight down, was the ocean.

As Sen had promised me, it was a most spectacular view. The steep walls of the mountain amplified the sounds of the waves far below, giving the illusion that the sea might have been only a stone's throw away. From this aerial view, somewhat magnified by a peculiar atmospheric distortion, one could watch the waves rolling gently in upon the beautiful white beach, appearing as they might through binoculars.

I was aware of Sen squatting down on the ledge a few feet off to my left and a foot or two behind me. I turned and watched as he took a small package from his daypack. He had something wrapped up in newspapers, which he set down in front of him.

He carefully unfolded the papers, smoothing the edges out over the ground. At the center of the square of newspaper were six objects that looked like green cactus apples with flattened tops. Each one had a feathery white tuft growing out of its top.

With a small, razor-sharp, stag handled jackknife, Sen removed the tufts and sliced the cactus apples pie-like into narrow wedges.

"What is it?" I asked, in Spanish.

"It is medicine for fixing your eyes," Sen said. He looked up and grinned mischievously, making a peculiar fanning gesture with his hands around the area of his eyes.

"Peyote," I said.

He nodded, inviting me to share the peyote with him.

I would have been reluctant except that back in the States, I had taken peyote three times. Each time had been under controlled conditions, and in the name of medical research. We had taken our peyote as a dried powder inside gelatin capsules. I had only seen pictures of it in its raw form.

I had experienced a pleasant, mildly altered state of consciousness in these experiments. So, naturally, I had no particular anxiety about taking the peyote with my guide.

Sen showed me how to eat the narrow slices from the buttons. He tipped back his head, opened his mouth wide, and placed a single slice far back on his tongue. Then he rocked his head forward and swallowed. On my first try, I failed to get the peyote far enough back on my tongue, and the foul, earthy taste made me wretch.

Sen repeated his instructions, and this time I got it right. Together we consumed five ripe buttons in about a half an hour. Then we sat quietly, breathing slowly and deeply in a way that Sen said he had been taught to do. I recall feeling nauseous at first, but had no trouble with it when I followed Sen's breathing instructions.

It was late evening. The sun was setting, and the sky had turned a deep scarlet. At the horizon, sea and sky blended as one in a symphony of reds and yellows.

Spread out between the ocean and the cave where we sat, I saw a strip of tropical jungle. Here was a world of lush greens, ferns and palms in varying tone, now wearing an aura of pink created by the fading sun.

Blowing in from the ocean, the evening air was cool, heavy with the earthy fragrance of the jungle, of naturally composting vegetation and moist soil, and of flowers which I could not see.

"It is like I told you it would be," Sen said. "Do you agree?"

I nodded, agreeing that indeed it was very beautiful.

Minutes passed; then Sen announced, "Darkness will be coming soon."

It took a moment for these words to sink in. And then the horror of it struck me. We had just spent the entire afternoon hiking up an extremely precipitous trail, along which we encountered many hazards. Several times I had clung to the rock face of the mountain to traverse a section of the trail washed out by storms, risking a fall of several hundred feet. Another time a large snake blocked the trail. Sen chased it off with a stick, all the while assuring me that the snake was not poisonous, though its bite could be harmful.

The realization that I might have to go down this same trail in the darkness startled me. How could I have been so stupid! Why had it not occurred to me, until now, that it would be dark when we returned!

I was furious with Sen. What sort of person would guide me to such a place, heedless of the threat to my well-being. Surely he realized it would be dark before we returned.

I then became aware of a deep, groaning roar coming from deep within the cave behind me, and I leapt to my feet with visions of being attacked at any moment by a wild animal whose peace we had disturbed. I began swearing and jumping around, unable to decide which way to turn. I knew there was a washout less than a hundred yards down the trail, and it was was already too dark to safely cross it.

Sen continued to sit at the mouth of the cave, completely unperturbed. In fact, he was wearing a toothy grin that did nothing for my sense of security.

Again I heard the groaning roar within the cave. "What the hell is that?" I cried. "Don't you think we should get out of here?"

"Is it such a bad sound?" Sen asked. "I find it rather pleasant."

"Pleasant!" I said, still searching for an escape. "How can you sit there so calmly? Do you know what it is?"

"It is a sound."

"Of what?"

Sen shrugged. "Who knows?"

At that moment, I sensed that he knew something which I didn't. He'd been here before. Or at least he claimed that he had been. He obviously knew that the sound wasn't a threat to our safety. Or did he? I knew nothing about the man, other than what I saw. He had told me nothing about himself. Where had he come from? For all I knew he cold be a complete fool, or a madman—some sort of murderer who lured people out into the wilds where he slaughtered them. After all, who would ever find me out here? Who even knew—or for that matter cared—where I'd gone?

"Sit down," he said sternly, pointing to the empty boulder at the mouth of the cave where moments before I had been sitting.

"Not on your life," I said.

He looked at me incredulously. "No? Then, where are you going to go?"

"I'm leaving," I said. "I'll go back down the trail."

"Surely you're joking."

"I'm not joking at all," I said. "I've had plenty of trail experience back in California.

"Suit yourself," he said. "But you'll miss the best part of the sunset. Look." He pointed over the horizon.

Against my better judgment I turned to find out what he thought could possibly be so important. At the edge of the horizon the sky was ablaze with a bright pattern of red and yellow light, twisting slowly into a shape that resembled a spiral galaxy. My breath was literally taken away by the beauty of it, and for a moment I completely forgot my plight.

"My god, what is it?" I asked.

"It is what I promised you," Sen said. "I have kept my word."

In spite of myself I sat down and stared out over the horizon. For an hour or more I watched as the spiraling colors played at the end of the ocean. The galaxy of colors was huge, awesome in its proportions, and seemed to have a life of its own, twisting and turning almost playfully, as though it had an intelligence and was performing a dance with the Earth.

Then suddenly it was gone, and we were plunged into darkness.

The groaning roar rose from the cave behind us, and this time I was able to study it, to listen with a calmer mind. Rather than like an animal, it sounded this time like two gigantic boulders being ground slowly together, emitting a voice from somewhere deep down in the earth beneath our feet. I had visions of two continental plates scraping against one another, their sound amplified and made more resonant by a long tunnel in the cave.

"Listen," Sen said. "Listen."

I did, and the sound varied, not like a voice so much as like music made by a gigantic instrument whose shape and mechanics I could barely imagine.

"Didn't I tell you?" Sen said excitedly. "Didn't I tell you I would show you a wonderful place?"

He leaned down and picked up his knapsack. Reaching inside, he produced a round object which he handed to me. It was too dark to see what it was, but from the size and texture I guessed it was an orange.

"Supper," Sen said, announcing this in a completely matter-of-fact tone.

Was he kidding? Was this really his idea of an adequate supper after our arduous climb to this place? Without comment, I sullenly peeled and sectioned the orange, determining that I would eat it slowly, savoring every bite.

I was aware of Sen rolling his orange between his palms, the peeling still in place. He was doing this in a very studied, very methodical way, and I grew curious. As I watched him, I also became aware that the mountain was growing brighter and brighter, almost as though a huge spotlight was being pointed at us. I looked up and saw the edge of a full moon just emerging from behind the top of the mountain, another five hundred feet above us. This was providing us with enough light to safely make our way down the path, if that is what we chose to do.

I looked at Sen, meaning to suggest this to him. But now he was ripping into the orange like a starving ape, tearing off great chunks and burying his face in his hands as he sucked and chewed at the fruit. I was disgusted by his behavior, and wondered if he always ate like this. He finished, reached into his knapsack for a bandanna, and wiped off his face and hands, licking his fingers now and then to get rid of the sticky juice. This done, he lay down, arranged the knapsack under his head, and appeared for all the world to be getting ready to take a nap.

"Shouldn't we be getting back while we still have some light from the moon?" I asked.

"What's the hurry? Have you got an appointment with the doctor or something?" To this he chuckled stupidly, like a man unaware of the fact that no one else thought his joke funny.

"When *are* we going back?"

"Why don't you just enjoy yourself," he said. "Take it easy."

I don't know whether I was more angry than anxious, but I could see that there was no sense in trying to budge him. He had his own plans for us, and he was obviously not going to let me in on them. I was completely at his mercy.

I leaned back and started picking at the orange that I had sectioned so carefully. I picked up the first section and was about to put it in my mouth when I felt something moving across my hand. I looked down at the orange section. A tiny lizard, about the length of my little finger, clung to the fruit. I grabbed it by the tail and flung it out into space, disgusted by the thought that had I not felt it moving in time, I would have bitten into it, and might at this very moment be spitting out its bleeding carcass.

I was careful after that, brushing off each section of fruit and inspecting it in the moonlight before popping it into my mouth. By the time I had finished eating, Sen was sound asleep. His rasping snores indicated to me that it would be no use trying to awaken him, at least not for an hour or more.

I felt restless and uneasy. From far below us I could hear waves lapping against the beach, and this was soothing. Then, every few minutes, the cave made that peculiar groaning sound, a sound to which I had now become accustomed. To pass the time, I decided that I would try to plot how long were the silences between the cave's groans, but after an hour or more I could determine no apparent pattern, and eventually gave it up.

The moonlight slowly faded, and again I became anxious as darkness closed in around me. Now, every sound seemed amplified, and I became aware of live things all around me. High-pitched whistles from inside the cave suggested the presence of bats. Rustling in the trees suggested night birds, or perhaps nocturnal animals. None of these things particularly disturbed me, though they didn't exactly put me at ease, either. I had spent many nights under the stars back in the States, hiking in the Sierras. But I have to admit that these sounds were not familiar to me, and my inability to identify them put my nerves on edge.

The sky was brilliant with stars, the Milky Way like a great sea of light. Several times I saw meteorites trailing across the sky. In spite of my nervousness, I caught myself dozing, jerking to attention when by body relaxed, and I almost lost the balance of my sitting position. At last I gave into it and lay down, staring up at the sky until I fell asleep.

The next thing I knew there was a shriek, and I sat bolt upright, not knowing what to expect. The shriek shattered the stillness once more and I looked up, having determined that the sound had come from above and to my left. As I searched the darkness, the shriek came again and a huge bird, with a wingspan of at least six feet, swooped down, coming right for me. I leapt behind Sen's rock— where he continued to sleep soundly—just as the great bird shot by.

As the bird passed, less than a foot from my face, I saw its talons extended as though for a kill. But that was not the worst of it. Just a few feet past me, it stopped in mid-flight, seemed to gather itself into a ball, and suddenly changed directions, facing me once again as thought preparing for another attack. I shielded my face with both arms, fully expecting to feel its sharp talons dig into me at any moment. But then it stopped. Facing me directly, flapping its wings gently, hanging in the air like a feathery helicopter, I thought I heard it make a sound.

Surely I was dreaming. But I knew I wasn't. I looked directly at the bird and saw that it had a human face. I rubbed my eyes, certain that what I was seeing couldn't possibly be true. But it was. The bird had a human face. Moreover, it was a face I recognized. It was Sen's face! Sen had taken the form of a giant night-hunter. I glanced down on the ground where he had been sleeping. Indeed, he was gone. And there, as clear as the paper on which these words are printed, was the bird—Sen in the form of a bird, hovering before my eyes, flapping his wings gently, evenly, as he held his space in the air.

"What are you doing?" I asked, at the moment not thinking how indescribably unbelievable it was to be talking to a bird who had taken the face of my companion.

"Coo! Coo! Coo!" the bird said. This was followed by laughter—laughter that I knew was Sen's. The laughter ended and was followed by his stupid chuckling. Did he somehow expect me to share in his little joke? I didn't think it was funny. In fact, I was shaking like a leaf, still unable to give a rational explanation for what I'd seen. Besides, the bird was still there, still hovering within an arm's length me.

I decided to treat it as an everyday occurrence. After all, maybe it was a dream. I had heard that the best way to stop a person or situation that you don't like in a dream was to rein in your rational self and tell it to go away. I did this, and heard the bird reply, "Go away to where? You said yourself, it wasn't safe to go down the trail in the dark."

"But you're a bird," I said. "You can fly."

"Oh, right. That's right," I heard Sen say. "Goo'bye, then."

And with this, he disappeared. By the light of the stars I watched him gather his wings under him and plunge off the cliff where I was sitting. I watched as he circled gracefully, changed direction, and disappeared, skimming the treetops in the jungle below, apparently continuing his night hunt.

Then, startled, I suddenly realized that I was all alone at the mouth of the cave. Could this have actually happened? Had Sen been transformed, somehow, into the body of a bird, a giant owl or whatever it was? In any case, it was very clear to me now that I was left alone on the mountainside.

I heard the crunch of gravel on the path a hundred feet away, off to my right. I called out, "Sen, is that you?"

Much to my relief, my companion came into view, hooking up his pants.

"Where were you?" I asked.

"I went to take a crap," he said. "What's wrong? Are you late for your appointment again?" This was followed by his usual stupid chuckle. Then he went back over to his rock and stretched out, arranging the knapsack under his head as before.

"I've had enough of this," I said. "Stop fooling around with my head."

"I'm going back to sleep," he said. "Wake me when the movie's over."

I could not believe his audacity or his incredible coolness. Within seconds he was sound asleep again, apparently oblivious to everything going on around him. I lay brooding, angry, thoroughly shaken by everything I had been through that night. I wanted to grab Sen by the shoulders and shake him awake. I wanted to scream at him, to tell him how much I resented the games he was playing with me. I didn't know how he was accomplishing what he was doing, and I didn't care. I just wanted it to stop.

I huddled close to my rock like an animal guarding its territory. I myself began to feel like an animal, destined to live out its life in the wild. I felt a warming sensation throughout my body, a rippling of muscle. Perhaps it was due to a warm breeze emitted from the mouth of the cave. It was certainly possible that there were hot springs somewhere below that occasionally emitted heat which escaped to the outer vestibules.

I found myself staring steadily and angrily at the sleeping Sen. I had never felt such hatred for another man. But as I stared at him I could not identify my anger. I felt a strange fear, like nothing I'd ever felt before. It was as though this man was an intruder in my life, that he was threatening me or something that belonged to me.

I watched him cautiously, waiting for him to make the slightest move in my direction, a move that would indicate that I would have to fight with him—perhaps until one or the other of us was dead. I determined that I would be the victor. After all, I was larger, more powerful than he.

Sen's snoring stopped. He took a deep breath, then suddenly began to tremble all over as though he was having some sort of fit. The light changed and I saw a giant cat, a mountain lion or a panther standing between me and him, teeth bared.

"Sen," I cried, wanting to warn him. But a strange sound came from my throat, a hissing that I could barely identify with.

Sen sat bolt upright and looked calmly past the cat. In fact, his gaze was piercing, looking right through the cat into my eyes. "Stop this nonsense right now," he said. "You need your sleep. You'll be exhausted in the morning."

"The cat," I said. "Don't you see it?" At that moment I wasn't certain of anything. I could not clearly see the cat myself. It was too close for me to see. I was terribly confused. Why couldn't he see it? I was aware only of its threatening posture, baring its teeth, ready to pounce.

"Of course I see it," Sen said. "It's your cat. It's not going to hurt me."

My cat, I thought to myself. *Mine?* And then I asked, "What makes you so sure?"

"I am just sure. I am just sure." He waved his hand in front of my face. Suddenly I was calm. I felt spellbound. "You see?" Sen said.

Sen lay back down, and in seconds he was sound asleep again. I drew back away from him, toward the mouth of the cave. The cat came back into focus for me. It was just me and the cat now. The cat turned, gazed into my face, and appeared to grin.

Was all this truly my own creation? I stared back at the cat. Its face lit up, glowing, as though it had been a plastic mask; now someone had turned on a light behind the cat mask, exposing the illusion. The body of the cat vanished and I was looking just at its face, at that backlit mask. Then the mask of the cat began to dissolve, as though the heat of the light behind it was causing it to melt. Soon it was nothing more than a molten blob turning in space like a star. As I watched, it began to reshape itself into a much more geometric form.

After a few moments its transformation was complete. Round, saucer-shaped, it turned slowly in the space before my eyes. The light still shown within it, as though it possessed its own source of illumination. It turned again and again, revealing its full configuration, thin and elliptical from the side, round and perfectly symmetrical from the front. It was a lens, like the lens from a telescope or a magnifying glass. But this lens had an organic appearance—not unlike a living cell, translucent and soft, definitely alive—a geometric jellyfish.

I moved closer to the lens. Deep inside it I saw movement. What were these shapes? I saw many images from my childhood—my brothers, the house where I'd lived during my high school years in Michigan, my parents, my first lover. I thought about how people often reported seeing their lives flash before their eyes when they were faced with death. Could this be the case? Was I near death? I looked deeper into the lens, as though I might find the answer there. I saw a cat, a powerful mountain lion. There was also a giant bird. There was a groaning cave, and a beautiful sunset over the ocean. There was a rugged trail up a mountain, and a man. I looked more closely. It was Sen. He was sleeping by the rock, his head on his knapsack. I could not figure out where he was—in the lens, or beyond it, or both?

The lens turned in the air. I closed my eyes, trying to block it out, trying to see around it, or to see a clear place through it where the world beyond would not be distorted by the images inside the lens. But I could not escape the lens' influence, and now I was aware that it was turning deep in my consciousness, in the same space out of which dream and imagination are created. I had never before noticed how large this mental space I called imagination could be. It had no limits, no beginning or middle or end. It seemed to stretch out in all directions, a vast landscape whose borders were as unlimited as space itself.

At one moment I could be on the mountainside with Sen, in Mexico. A second later I was back in Michigan, many years before, a boy of twelve riding his bicycle on a rainslick asphalt street. A second after that I was driving across the Arizona desert in January, with a carload of friends, all in our early twenties, heading back to

California after a Christmas holiday with our families in Michigan. Now I shifted to a backpacking trip in the high Sierras, where I fished for trout on the bank of a mountain lake.

Where was the lens now? I couldn't find it. It seemed to have merged with all the rest, lost in the jumble of everything I held in my consciousness. I felt panic. Losing the image of the lens was like losing a treasure I had dreamed of discovering all my life. Then there was a long moment of perfect clarity when I realized what had happened to the lens. I saw that it hadn't disappeared at all; the lens was my consciousness, not simply a piece of it.

For a long time I just sat quietly and thought about this. It seemed to me that the lens was like a vehicle for my awareness, giving me an identity separate from the rest of the world. This was the image I had been seeking since I was a child. A thousand questions and speculations that I had entertained along the way now focused on this lens image.

Having the sense of separateness which the lens provided seemed to me both exciting and frightening. It meant that I was not like an ant, with instincts—that is, pre-programmed responses built in—dictating my every action. It meant that I was capable of creating my own program, or even of overriding whatever biological or God-given programs might be built in.

My decisions, my fears, my dreams, my acquired knowledge, all could come into play. In my present situation, up on the mountain, I could make a decision, based on my fears or on other factors contained in my lens, to leave my guide sleeping by the mouth of the cave and make my way down the mountain trail alone. Or I could choose to trust him, and wait for morning. Regardless of which decision I made, because of my awareness of my separateness—achieved through the lens—it was now very clear to me that I alone was responsible for my destiny. I was terribly excited about being able to see all this. This vision of the lens provided me with a symbol for making sense of knowledge I hadn't even been aware that I was collecting over the years. I wanted to awaken Sen and discuss it all with him.

"Sen," I said. "Sen, are you asleep?" I went over to him and gently shook his shoulder.

"What do you want?" he asked, turning his head to face me. "Have you created another cat? A bird?"

I started to look for the words to explain what I was seeing. But then I backed away. I realized that Sen already knew about everything I had seen. To him it was common knowledge, and he had no time for it. "Never mind," I said, deeply hurt by the realization that I had no one with whom to share my discovery. "I'm sorry to disturb you."

Sen mumbled something I couldn't understand and went back to sleep.

I sat down and watched the world beyond the lens, and saw it all merge with memories, images, ideas and feelings that I knew belonged only to me.

As my companion slept, the shadows shortened on the ledge where I sat and I saw that the lens was not something new in my life. I saw it far more clearly than ever before, and *that part* was new and unfamiliar, but the subtle mergings of external sights, sounds, sensations, all seemed normal, automatic, even familiar to me. I realized that these things had always occurred—and the only difference was that now I could see them, could feel their shifts and mergings, their constant metamorphoses from one form to another.

I remembered many times in the past, all through my life, when I had also had brief glimpses into these basic truths about our ways of processing reality, glimpses never more substantial than the sun's reflection from a bright chrome strip on a passing car. I now saw why life really was not all it appeared to be. Rather, it took on meaning only as it merged with our images inside the lens.

Later that afternoon, as we made our way back down the mountain, Sen listened patiently as I related the story of what had happened to me up on the mountain. I wanted to know if he had experienced any of it. Were the things I had seen a shared reality? Had he seen any of it?

Sen shrugged. He was vague and elusive. He told me that the Indians believed that the place where we spent the night was a *sacred spot* , and that people often had visions there that changed their lives. I asked if he had ever had visions there.

"Oh, yes," he said. "That is why I sleep when I go there. When I sleep it does what it must do and I am not always jumping up and down thinking I have to do something about it." He laughed. "Unlike you, I am a very lazy man."

When I tried to get him to explain this to me, he said it wasn't important. He told me my Spanish wasn't good enough to understand him if he really tried to go into it. And his English wasn't good enough for him to even attempt it in my language.

He dismissed me with that phrase the Mexicans have for stopping all further conversation on a subject: *"No me importa"*—it is not important to me. "You went to the mountain and you saw what I promised you. I am a very good guide. I hope you will tell your friends about me."

I promised him I would.

When I got back to the camp where I was staying, Sen disappeared down the beach and I never saw him again. I asked the owner of the hostel about him, and he told me that Sen was an Indian, and that I was lucky to have come back from the trek at all. Sen belonged to a tribe that still lived in the mountains, and they were not known for their friendliness toward Anglos. They had no respect at all for the laws of the Government, and they lived their lives completely cut off from the rest of the world.

I always took this warning with a grain of salt. After all, if Sen's people were so isolated from the rest of civilization, how had he learned English? He knew my language far better than I knew his. Moreover, when I thought back on it I could not think of a single incident in which Sen had acted in any way that I considered directly harmful. Any harm that could have come to me would have come from my own lens distorting reality in ways that could have caused me to use bad judgment and perhaps bring me to harm through my own actions.

The experience has stayed with me throughout my life and become something far more than an unusual memory. The lens has become a reference point for me, a kind of metaphor over which I have puzzled for many years. Only in the past couple years has it become comfortable for me to write about it, to relate the story to others so that I might share the revelations that have come from it.

—Hal Zina Bennett

THE LENS OF PERCEPTION by Hal Zena Bennett, 1987. Courtesy of *SHAMAN'S DRUM, A Journal Of Experiential Shamanism*: Fall, 1987

Letters To The Editor

Dear Mr. Mount:

Thank you for sending *The Peyote Book* which I read with a great deal of interest. Had I known the nature of the soil and the amount of light required, I might still have my peyote plant. I believed that it did not respond, because I smothered it with TLC. I kept it in a flower pot in a south window and watered it regularly like any other plant. The wonder is that it lived at all.

When I moved to Arizona, I planted it under a Carub tree and paid little attention to it. Since my Arapaho friends had described the beauty of the blossoms, I was delighted to see it flourish and bloom. I had to keep it covered with a strawberry box (open-mesh plastic) to keep the rabbits from devouring it.

The environment agreed with it, so I left it there when I returned to Wyoming to live. After some twenty years, I still have the dried button my friends gave me when I was doing field work at Wind River for my ethnography, *The Arapahoes, Our People.*

—Virginia C. Trenholm,
Author & Historian

Dear Friends:

I just read Guy Mount's book on Native Medicine, and totally devoured the book in one day. My personal experience with peyote was similar to Guy's. It works best with prayer, a humble surrender and focused meditation.

—Savitri, Registered Massage Therapist

More Letters

Dear Friends:

I was appalled last night when I turned on the news to hear that the U.S. Supreme Court had ruled against [our Constitutional] right to use peyote as a religious sacrament...Half a century of scientific studies have shown that peyote is a non-addictive, mildly psychoactive plant...The court has reversed existing federal laws that specifically permitted American Indian use of peyote, thus antagonizing one quarter million Native American Church members. Yet in the 1960 case of Mary Attakai, the court once said:

> "The manner in which peyote is used by the Indian worshipper is not inconsistent with public health, morals or welfare. Its use...is in fact entirely consistent with the good morals, health and spiritual elevation of some 225,000 Indians."

Native American Church practitioners adamantly believe peyote is not a drug, but an herbal medicine and spiritual sacrament. They are equally adamant that peyote should never be mixed with alcohol or drugs. In fact the NAC has been more successful in helping Indians overcome their drug and alcohol dependencies than any other organization. When alcohol was outlawed during the 1930s, the National Prohibition Act (18th Amendment) specifically exempted wine used for sacramental purposes. Peyote has been used by Native people for thousands of years. Does the U.S. Constitution only recognize Christian sacraments?

A variety of religious traditions were supposed to be guaranteed protection by the Constitution, yet many Native American religions have been held in the deepest contempt by this ruling because they do not measure up to the definitions of religion as laid down by European ideas of what constitutes a sacrament...How can we turn our backs on the people and religion which most reveres this land?

—Maria, California

To The Editor

Hello:

My Family and I have been seekers of spiritual experience for over twenty years. We have meditated, fasted, yoga'd and read spiritual books until our eyes turned red. Certainly these pursuits have been worthwhile; but honestly, the only real touches I have had with the spirit have been the three times I have used the sacrament peyote. Visions, tears, ecstasy and many valuable lessons were experienced. I felt kinship with the spirit beyond space and time, as well as kinship with other peyote worshippers in the past, present and future. Peyote was indeed a very significant religious sacrament for me. I believe our right to religious freedom must be preserved.

I miss the peyote way of worshipping, and I wish I could continue it with my family. Fear of oppression prevents my religious expression...A legalized access to peyote for personal religious use would be a wonderful coloring to life in the shadows.

—George, Montana

Happy Earth Day!

Well it is almost inconceivable that the U.S. Supreme Court, against the tide of scholarly opinion, should rule against [federal protection for] the use of peyote in religious ceremonies. But I suppose in the growth of any complex civilization there comes a time when control of human activity becomes more important to the state than the ideological or moral principals upon which that society was founded.

Surely our constitutional right to freedom of religion, granted to us by the founding fathers of our nation, is more worthy of protection that a criminal code passed in the last few decades that makes an uninformed classification of peyote as a dangerous drug. It is clear that we must defend our position and the constitution now, lest peyotism goes the way of the wolf and buffalo in America's attempt to dominate or destroy all that is natural and free-roaming.

—Randy, Maryland

More Feedback

Dear Editor:

The American Indian has consistently had to fight for his religious right to use the peyote cactus, a completely unaddictive psychoactive drug basic to a [religion] that has done wonders against alcoholism and other problems, and for self-respect among American Indians throughout the Native American Church. Some of our western and southwestern states have enacted oppressive laws against the...use of peyote, quite against Federal laws that permit its ceremonial use.

[The Peyote Book] should be had by anyone interested in the ethnobotany of peyote and in the rights of a true minority to practice their own unoffensive religion based on an inoffensive plant.

—Professor Richard E. Schultes
Director Botanical Museum
Harvard University

Dear Friends:

Regarding the recent Supreme Court case involving the state of Oregon...I believe the state is trying to divert attention from its inability to eradicate drug abuse. Peyote is certainly not to blame for drug abuse and neither is marijuana or any other plant. Drug abuse starts and ends with people who simply forget—or never learn—that they are a part of the Great Spirit or life force. The connection between the source of life and its many manifestation is ignored. A foolish selfishness rules and any number of substances become more important than honoring, praising and thanking the Great Spirit. I'm saying the true root cause of drug abuse is always spiritual. [And so is the solution—Editor.]

With Love and Respect
—Leo, New York

A Book Review

The public hysteria surrounding the federal government's so-called "War on Drugs" has had a profound impact on America's Indian Communities. Since The first contacts with Europeans nearly five centuries ago, Indians have had to brace themselves against assaults on their cultures, religions, and way of life. Now their religious freedom is under renewed attack because the U.S. Supreme Court has ruled that the Constitution does not exempt people from complying with state laws regarding the use of peyote. This decision allowed the state of Oregon to deny unemployment benefits to two men who had used peyote in ceremonies of the Native American Church. Ironically, the men had been counselors in a state-funded drug rehabilitation program.

In recent years, calls for strict punishment of all drug users have intensified. But while the use of peyote for religious purposes is protected under federal law—the American Indian Religious Freedom Act of 1978—the danger remains that peyote may be lumped with illegal drugs in the eyes of the public. Few Americans are aware that the small peyote cactus, a nonaddictive hallucinogen, has long been used by Indians for medicinal and religious purposes. For this reason, education—spreading the truth about peyote—is important; popular books and articles that describe the cactus and how Indians have used it historically can help reduce the public's growing anxiety toward peyote and the Native American Church. Guy Mount's *The Peyote Book: A Study of Native Medicine* [is an] attempt to provide part of that education.

Although there is already an extensive literature describing peyote and its use, many of the books and articles are oriented toward scholars and graduate students. Edward F. Anderson's *Peyote, The Divine Cactus* ranks among the best of these studies. The popular literature, while rather extensive, has often presented a muddled view of peyote and has rarely described its history in a comprehensive fashion. Among the few good popular accounts is Alice Marriott's and Carol K. Rachlin's *Peyote*, published in 1971.

Like Marriott and Rachlin, Guy Mount gives the general reader insight into the "legends, healing testimonials, spiritual and philosophical perceptions, songs, stories and artwork inspired by the Good Medicine." Mixing excerpts from the works of Anderson, Virginia Trenholm, Vine Deloria, James Slotkin, Virgil Vogel, [Omer Stewart] and others, with Indian narratives and stories as well as his own poetry and writing, Mount offers an entertaining picture of peyote history. His brief volume includes Yaqui, Apache, and Shoshone peyote origin stories; healing stories; accounts by Indian women on how peyote facilitates childbirth; insights into the gathering and cultivation of the cactus; scientific and medical investigations into its medicinal uses; and various descriptions of the Native American Church. A legal section examines the complexities of the federal and state legal systems as they apply to peyote.

Readers interested in a broad perspective and a written introduction to peyote's mysteries are well served by Guy Mount's *Peyote Book*.

—Joseph B. Herring
National Archives
Washington, D.C.

The American Indian Quarterly: Fall,1991.
University of California, Native American Studies Dept., Berkeley.

About The Editor

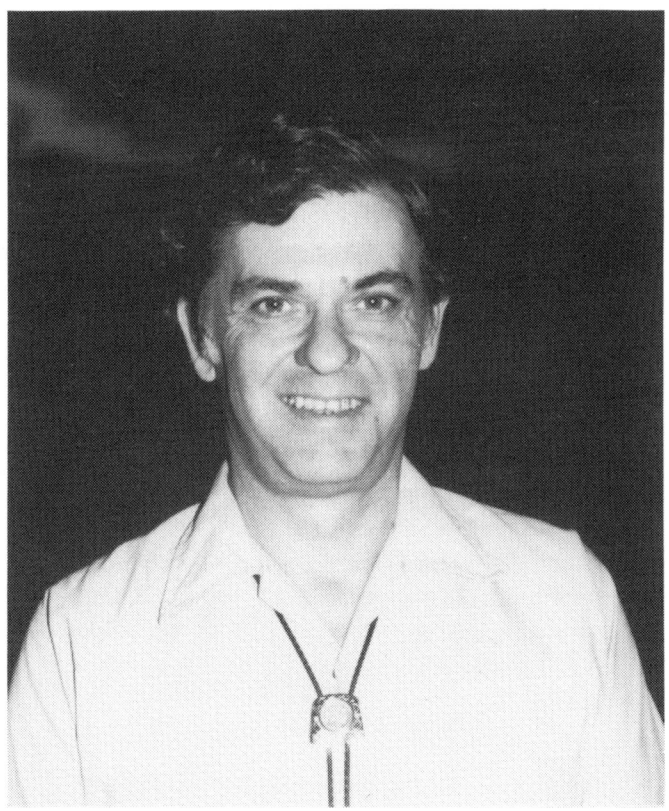

Guy Mount has a Master's Degree in Educational Anthropology with California Teaching Credentials. He has taught Native American Studies on a High School and College level, and has been a student of Native American medicine, philosophy and religion since 1968. Publications include *Not For Innocent Ears, The Peyote Book, Coyote's Big Penis and Other Stories.*

Guy describes his own ethnic ancestry as "all mixed up." He proudly calls himself an "earthperson," meaning someone who finds their identity in the earth, rather than an empire. "You see," he explains, "The challenge for everyone is to become an earthperson, regardless of their ethnic heritage. Mother Earth needs our help to survive. Also, a personal identity based on one's position in an empire may prove shallow and self-destructive. Whereas Mother Earth will always love us, no matter how old we get. Our job is to help renew the earth, to ask ourselves: what have I done for the medicine today? What can I do for our mother? Some days I just walk in the woods and plant acorns. It's a challenge to be an earthperson. But it's the best job around. Mother Earth is an excellent employer."

Bibliography

Aberle, David F.
1966

The Peyote Religion Among The Navaho. Aldine Publishing: Chicago.

Achendel, Gordon
1968

Medicine In Mexico, From Aztec Herbs To Betatrons. University of Texas, Austin.

Anderson, E.F.
1960

"The Biogeography, Ecology, and Taxonomy of *Lophophora* (Cactacea)," *Brittonia.* XXI, 299-310.

1980

Peyote, The Divine Cactus. University of Arizona Press: Tucson

Andrews, Edmund
1903

"The Aboriginal Physicians of Aboriginal Michigan," *Contributions to Medical Research.* George Wahr, pgs. 42-50, Ann Arbor.

Artaud, A.
1976

The Peyote Dance. Translated from French by Helen Weaver. Farrar, Straus and Giroux: New York.

Bass, Althea
1966

The Arapaho Way. Clarkson N. Potter: New York.

Benitez, Fernando
1968

En La Tierra Magica del Peyote. Biblioteca Era, Mexico.

Bennett, Hal Z.
1987

The Lens Of Perception. Celestial Arts: Berkeley, CA.

Bennett, W.C., and
Zingg, R.M.
1936

The Tarahumara, An Indian Tribe Of Northern Mexico. University of Chicago Press: Chicago.

Bergman, Robert L.
1971

"Navaho Peyote Use—Its Apparent Safety," *American Journal Of Psychiatry.* 12/71.

Boke, N. H. and
Anderson, E.F.
1970.

"Structure, Development and Taxonomy in the Genus, *Lophophora*," *American Journal Of Botany.* LVII, 5, 569-78.

Boyd, Doug
1975

Rolling Thunder. Random House: New York.

Brandon
1971

The Magic World, American Indian Songs and Poems. Wm. Morrow: New York.

Brandt, W.
and C. Tranter
1943

"Peyote Intoxication: Some Psychological Aspects Of The Peyote Rite," *Journal Of Nervous And Mental Disorders.* V97:518.

Brito, Silvester
1989

The Way Of A Peyote Roadman. Peter Lang Publishing: New York.

Castaneda, Carlos
1968

The Teachings Of Don Juan. Ballantine Books: New York.

1971

A Separate Reality. Simon & Shuster: New York.

Chidamian, Claude
1958

The Book Of Cacti And Other Succulents. Doubleday: New York.

Crow Dog
1971

Crow Dog's Paradise: Songs Of The Sioux. Electra Records: New York. Featuring singers Henry and Leonard Crow Dog with Leonard Running on water drum.

D'Azevedo, Warren L.
1978

Straight With The Medicine. Heyday Books: Berkely, CA.

Deloria, Vine
1969

Custer Died For Your Sins. Macmillian Publishing: New York.

Der Marderosian, A.
1965

"Current Status Of Hallucinogens In The Cactaceae," *American Journal Of Pharmacy.* CXXXVIII,204-12.

Dorrance, D.
et. al.
1975

"Effect Of Peyote On Human Chromosones." *Journal Of The American Medical Assosciation.* Vol. 234, No. 3:299-302.

Ellis, Havelock
1902

"Mescal, A Study Of A Divine Plant," *Popular Science Monthly.* 41:52-71.

1898   "Mescal, A New Artificial Paradise," *Annual Report Of The Smithsonian Institution.* Washington DC: 537-48.

Feder, Norman   *American Indian Art.* Abrams: New York.
1965

Flattery, D.   *Peyote.* Berkeley Press: Berkeley, CA.
and J. Pierce
1965

Furst, Peter T.   "Huichol Conceptions Of The Soul,"
1967   *Folklore Americas.* XXVII, 2, 39-106.

1971   "*Ariocarpus retusus,* The 'False Peyote' Of Huichol Tradition," *Economic Botany.* XXV, 182-87.

1972   *Flesh Of The Gods.* "To Find Our Life: Peyote Among The Huichol Indians Of Mexico." Praeger: New York.

Gaskin, Stephan   *The Caravan.* Book Publishing Co.
no date   The Farm: Box 180, Summertown, TN.

no date   *Hey Beatnik.* Book Publishing Co.

Guerra, Francisco   *Libellus de Medicanalilus Indorum*
1952   *Herbius, El Manuscripto Pictorico Mexicano-Latino de Martin de la Cruz y Juan Badino de 1152.* Editorial: Vargas Rea Y El Diario Espanol. [Aztec Herbal] Available through Stanford Medical Research Library.

Hammerschlag, Carl   *The Dancing Healers, A Doctor's Journey*
1988   *Of Healing With Native Americans.* Harper & Row: San Francisco, CA.

Hamilton, Charles   *Cry Of The Thunderbird.* University of 1934,
New Ed. '72   Oklahoma Press: Norman, OK.

Herring, Joseph   "Book Review," **American Indian Quarterly:**
1991   U.C. Berkeley, NAS.

Huxley, Aldous   **The Doors Of Perception.** Harper and Row:
1954   New York.

Kapadia, G.J.   "Peyote Alkaloids," **Journal Of Pharma-**
1968   **cology Science.** 57:191-92 and 254-62.

Kelly, Isabel   **Folk Practices In North Mexico.** University
1965   of Texas Press: Austin, TX.

Kelsey, F.E.   "The Pharmacology Of Peyote," **South**
1959   **Dakota Journal Of Medicine.** 12:6, 231-33.

Kluver, Heinrich   **Mescal—The Divine Plant And Its**
1928   **Psychological Effects.** Paul, Trench,
                       Trubner & Company: London, England.

Knauer, A. and   "A Preliminary Note On The Psychic Action Of
W. Malone   Mescaline, With Special Reference To The
1913   Mechanisms Of Visual Hallucinations,"
                       Journal Of Nervous And Mental
                       Disorders. 40: 397-425.

LaBarre, W. and   "Statement On Peyote," **Science.** 114:582.
D.P. McAlister,
J.S. Slotkin,
O.C. Stewart,
Sol Tax.
1951

1969   **The Peyote Cult.** Revised and Augmented
                       Edition. University of Oklahoma: Norman.

Lame Deer, John and   **Lame Deer, Seeker of Visions: The Life**
Richard Erodes   **Of A Sious Medicine Man.** Simon and
1972   Schuster: New York.

Libhart, Miles, Ed.   **Contemporary Southern Plains Indian**
1972   **Painting.** Oklahoma Indian Arts and Crafts
                       Cooperative Press: Anadarko, OK.

Lundstom, Jan and   "Thin-layer Chromatography Of The Peyote
Augurell, Stig   Alkloids," **Journal Of Chromatography.**
1967   XXX, 271-72.

Lurie, Nancy O.   *Mountain Wolf Woman: The Auto-*
1966   *biography Of A Winnebago Indian*
                        Woman. The University of Michigan Press:
                        Ann Arbor.

Marriott, Alice   *Metal Jewelry Of The Peyote Cult.*
1942   Denver Art Museum: Denver.

1945   *The Ten Grandmothers.* "Peyote Way Of
                        Quanah Parker," Univ. of Oklahoma Press

and Carol Rachlin   *American Indian Mythology.* Thomas Y.
1968   Crowell Company: New York.

and Carol Rachlin   *Peyote.* Crowell: New York
1971

McAllester, D.P.   *Peyote Music.* Viking Fund, Publications In
1949   Anthropology: New York.

Mitchell, S. Weir   "The Effects Of Anhalonium Lewinii, (the mes-
1896   cal button)," *British Medical Journal.* 2:1625.

Momaday, N. Scott   *The Way To Rainy Mountain.* University
1969   of New Mexico Press: Albequerque.

1966   *House Made Of Dawn.* Harper & Row:
                        New York.

Mooney, James   *The Ghost Dance Religion.* Government
1896   Printing Office (Fourteenth Annual Report
                        of the Bureau of Ethnology.) Washington,D.C

Myerhoff, Barbara   "The Deer-Maize-Peyote Complex Among The
1968   Huichol Indians Of Mexico," Unpub. PhD Diss.
                        UCLA (Available on University Microfilms:
                        Ann Arbor.

1972   *The Peyote Hunt.* Cornell University Press:
                        Ithica, New York.

Opler, Morris E.   ***Apache Odyssey.*** Rinehart and Winston:
1969   New York.

Osol, Arthur, Ed.   ***The Dispensatory Of The United States,***
1955   ***25th Edition.*** Lippincott: Philadelphia.

Ott, J.   ***Hallucinogenic Plants Of North America.***
1976   Revised Ed. 1979, Wingbow Press: Berkeley.

Pennington, C.   ***The Tepehuan Of Chichuahua, Their***
1969   ***Material Culture.*** University of Utah Press:
                     Salt Lake City.

Pennington, C. W.   ***The Tarahumara Of Mexico, Their***
1963   ***Environment And Material Culture.***
                     University of Utah Press: Salt Lake City

Radin, Paul   ***The Autobiography Of A Winnebago***
1920   ***Indian.*** UC Pub.Am. Arch. & Ethn., 16:7
                     Dover Pub., 1963: New York.

Roseman, Bernard   ***The Peyote Story.***Wilshire Book Company:
1972   North Hollywood, Ca.

Rouhier, A,   ***Le Peyotl.*** Doin et Cix: Paris
1927

Safford, W.E.   "Peyote, The Narcotic Mescal Button Of The
1921   Indians," ***Journal of the American Medical***
                     Association. LXXVII, 1278-79.

Sahgun, Fray   ***The Florentine Codex, A General***
1950-63   ***History Of The THings Of New Spain.***
                     Translated by Anderson and Dibble. The
                     School of American Research and The
                     University of Utah: Santa Fe, NM.

Schultes, Richard   "Peyote (*Lophophora Williamsii Lemaire*
1937   *Coulter)And Its Uses,*" Unpublished PhD
                     Diss. Harvard University: Cambridge.

1940   "The Aboriginal Therapeutic Use Of
                            Lophophora Williamsii," **Cactus And
                            Succulent Journal.** XII

1948   "The Appeal Of Peyote (*LophophoraWilliamsii)*
                            As A Medicine," **American Anthropologist.**
                            XL, 698-715.

and A. Hoffman   **The Botany And Chemistry Of
                            Hallucinogens.** Springfield, Illinois.

1972   "An Overview Of Hallucinogens In The West
                            ern Hemisphere," **Flesh Of The Gods.** Edited
                            by Peter T. Furst. Praeger: New York.

and A. Hoffman   **Plants Of The Gods.** McGraw-Hill: England.
1979

Schonle, Ruth   "Peyote, The Giver Of Visions," **American
1925   Anthropologist.** XXVII, 53-75.

Slotkin, J.S.   "Menomini Peyotism," **American
                            Philosophical Society.** 42: 565-700.

1955   "The Peyote Way," **Tommorrow.** OV,3,64-701

1956.   **The Peyote Religion.** The Free Press:
                            Glencoe, Illinois.

Sun Bear, et .al.   **The Path With Power.** Prentice Hall:
1987   New York.

Stenburg, Molly P.   "The Peyote Cult Among Wyoming Indians,"
1945   **Western Archives.** University of Wyoming
                            Library: Laramie, WY.

Stewart, Omer C.   **The Peyote Religion: A History.**
1987   University of Oklahoma Press: Norman, OK.

Steinmetz, Paul B.   **Pipe, Bible, And Peyote Among The
1990   Oglala Lakota.** University of Tennessee
                            Press: Knoxville, TN.

Sturtevant, F.M.
and V.A. Drill
1956

"Effects of Mescaline In Laboratory Animals And The Influence Of Ataraxics On Mescaline Response," *Proceedings Of The Society Of Experimental Biology And Medicine.* 92:383.

Trenholm, Virginia
and M. Carley
Norman, OK.

The Shoshonis, Sentinals Of The Rockies. University of Oklahoma Press: 1964

1970

The Arapahoes, Our People. University of Oklahoma Press.

Urbina, Manuel

"El Peyote y El Ololiuque," *Anales del Museo Nacional.* VII, 25-38, Mexico City.

Walkington, David

"Antibiotic Activity Of An Extract Of Peyote," *Economic Botany.* 14:3. July-Sept.

Vestal, Paul
and R. Schultes
1939

The Economic Botany Of The Kiowa Indians . Botanical Museum Of Harvard University: Cambridge, MA.

Willoya, William
and V. Brown
1962

Warriors Of The Rainbow. Naturegraph Publishing: Happy Camp, CA .

Vogel, Virgil
1970

American Indian Medicine. University of Oklahoma Press: Norman, OK.

Indian Rights Manual Available

Lawyers who represent Indian tribes or tribal members on natural resources protection, archaeological protection, and sacred places, and religious freedom cases may find the *Manual For Protecting Indian Natural Resources* to be of great value. Part 1 discusses federal and tribal law; and Part 2 discloses ways to make effective arguments for Indian causes. The manual is available for $25 from the Native American Rights Fund, 1506 Broadway, Boulder, CO 80302.

—Courtesy **SHAMAN'S DRUM**
Spring 1987 Issue

Distributed Titles

The following list of books-in-print are related to the Peyote Religion. They can be ordered by mail from SWEETLIGHT BOOKS.

Custer Died For Your Sins by Vine Deloria   **$8.95**
University of Oklahoma: 278 pages, 1969.

Dancing Healers by Carl Hammerschlag   **$8.95**
Harper & Row: 170 pages, 1988.

House Made Of Dawn by N. Scott Momaday   **$7.95**
Harper & Row: 192 pages, 1966.

Lame Deer: Seeker of Visions by Richard Erdoes   **$4.95**
Pocketbooks: 278 pages, 1972.

Path Of Power by Sun Bear   **$9.95**
Prentice Hall: 232 pages, 1987.

Peyote, The Divine Cactus by E.F. Anderson   **$10.95**
University of Arizona: 248 pages, 1980.

Peyote Cult by Weston LaBarre   **$14.95**
University of Oklahoma: 334 pages, Enlarged 1989.

Peyote Religion: A History by Omer Stewart   **$29.95**
University of Oklahoma: 454 pages, Hardbound, 1987.

Pipe, Bible, And Peyote by Paul Steinmetz   **$29.95**
University of Tennessee: 296 pages, Hardbound, 1989.

Plants of the Gods by Richard E. Schultes   **$19.95**
Inner Traditions: 192 pages, Color Illustrations, 1979.

Rolling Thunder by Doug Boyd   **$9.95**
Dell Publishers, 288 pages, 1974.

Straight With The Medicine by W.L. d'Azevedo   **$5.95**
Heyday Books: 74 pages, 1978.

Sweetlight Books
16625 Heitman Road
Cottonwood, CA 96022

Published Titles

NOT FOR INNOCENT EARS $9.95
Spiritual Traditions Of A Desert Cahuilla Medicine Woman
By Ruby Modesto and Guy Mount, Revised Edition, 1986.
ISBN: 0-9604462-0-6

THE PEYOTE BOOK $9.95
A Study Of Native Medicine
Compiled and Edited by Guy Mount, 3rd Edition, 1993.
Illustrations and Bibliography
ISBN: 0-9604462-3-0

CANYON de CHELLY $8.95
The Timeless Fold
By Conger Beasley, Jr. 1988.
Photography by Mary S. Watkins
ISBN: 0-9604462-4-9

LADY OCEAN $2.95
A Love Story For Children
By Guy Mount, 1986.
Illustrations by Kitty Roach
ISBN: 0-9604462-2-2

COYOTE'S BIG PENIS $5.95
And Other Stories
By Guy Mount, 1989.
ISBN: 0-9604462-5-7

THE MARIJUANA MYSTERY $9.95
By Guy Mount, 1993.
ISBN: 0-9604462-8-1

To order by mail: send your name and address with a check or money order for the amount of each book desired—California residents add 7% sales tax—plus $1.05 for bookrate postage.

QUALITY BOOKS FOR PEOPLE WHO LOVE THE EARTH

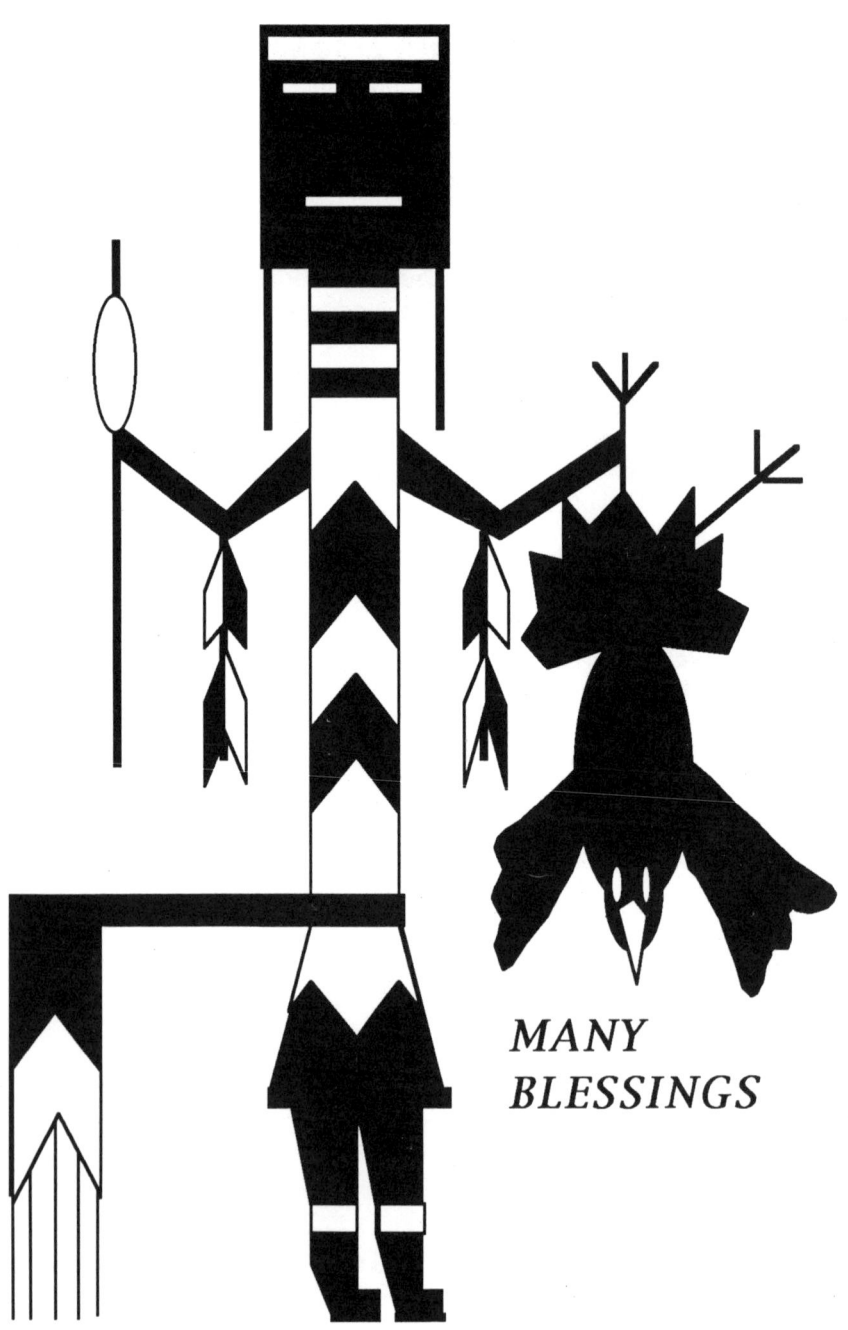

MANY
BLESSINGS

Artwork by Ruby